THE WORKBOOK *TO ACCOMPANY*

MOSBY'S CLINICAL DECISION VIDEO SERIES

FOR RESPIRATORY CARE

THE WORKBOOK *TO ACCOMPANY*
MOSBY'S CLINICAL DECISION VIDEO SERIES
FOR RESPIRATORY CARE

Patricia Fuchs Carroll, MS, RRT, RN
Owner
Educational Medical Consultants
Middletown, Connecticut
Adjunct Faculty, Respiratory Care
Manchester Community-Technical College
Manchester, Connecticut

Karen A. Milikowski, MS, RRT
Coordinator, Allied Health
Program Director, Respiratory Care
Manchester Community-Technical College
Manchester, Connecticut

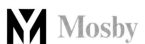

St. Louis Baltimore Boston Carlsbad Chicago Naples New York Philadelphia Portland
London Madrid Mexico City Singapore Sydney Tokyo Toronto Wiesbaden

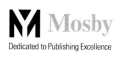

Dedicated to Publishing Excellence

A Times Mirror
Company

Publisher: Don Ladig
Editor: Jennifer Roche
Developmental Editor: Anne Gleason
Project Manager: Gayle Morris
Production Editor: Gina Keckritz
Layout Artist: Ken Wendling
Design Supervisor: Guy Jacobs
Cover Design: GW Graphics & Publishing, Inc.

Printed in the United States of America
Composition by Wordbench

Mosby-Year Book, Inc.
11830 Westline Industrial Drive
St. Louis, Missouri 63146

ISBN:0-8151-1474-5

96 97 98 99 00 / 9 8 7 6 5 4 3 2 1

Dedication

This video and workbook series is dedicated to:

Carl P. Wiezalis, RRT, MS

Carl Wiezalis was the program director when we attended the respiratory therapy program at the SUNY-Upstate Medical Center in Syracuse, New York twenty years ago, and he continues to lead the program into the future today. He was our first professional role model, and the values he instilled in us by his example are the cornerstone of our practice to this day.

Our commitment to the development of this series to help respiratory care practitioners develop clinical decision-making skills is a direct result of his lasting influence.

PFC
KAM

Acknowledgments

The success of a massive undertaking such as producing this video and workbook series is the result of a collaboration among a number of dedicated people.

Denny Hare, formerly of American Safety Video Publishers, encouraged me to pursue this concept for respiratory care and provided valuable feedback when the project was in its germinal stages.

Jim Shanahan, Mosby's respiratory care editor at the beginning of this project, considered and then championed the proposal and shared my vision for how these videos and this workbook could help respiratory care students and practitioners learn these important skills.

Anne Gleason, our developmental editor, gave us a crash course in publishing and kept this project on schedule. Her good humor, assistance, and guidance were invaluable.

Stan Lindsey, owner of Stan Lindsey Photography, Inc. in Naples, Florida was the still photographer for our cases. Even when it was late and we were exhausted, Stan persevered to make sure each shot was right.

The program reviewers, particularly Tim Op't Holt, provided us with thoughtful comments that helped us clarify ideas for our viewers and readers. They made a very positive contribution.

The manufacturers we contacted for equipment to use in the videos were very helpful. Special thanks to Pamela Ross, marketing manager for mechanical ventilation at Baxter Healthcare Corporation; and Monica Stevenson, marketing communications manager at Ohmeda, Inc.

Karen Milikowski, my coauthor and technical advisor, has been a friend and colleague since we lived across the hall from each other as respiratory therapy students twenty years ago. Her contributions during the writing, shooting, and editing of this project have consistently improved the finished product. Her support during the inevitable frustrations of such a complex venture helped keep me on track. Karen's obvious dedication to her students and the field of respiratory care education are a constant inspiration to me.

And, finally, to my husband, Bob, who was the glue that held this project together for me—from his late-night trips to pick me up at the airport in snowstorms to the gourmet dinners he prepared when I was in the office all day and almost all night; for sending that last-minute fax and for listening to me when I needed to vent (and resisting that insatiable urge to say "I told you so")—I don't know what I would do without him. Now, if he could only teach our dogs how to run the copier . . . .

To all of you, a heartfelt thanks.

PFC

I would like to express my sincere gratitude to the following people:

Patricia Fuchs Carroll, a brilliant and kindhearted person who I have admired since our college days at "Upstate Medical." Thank you for sharing your vision with me.

My family, who let me disappear from their lives for the past year.

Kerry Jean Connor, for her generous support and flexibility. Without it, I could not have been involved in such a wonderful and challenging project.

Eleanor Weseloh and Manchester Community-Technical College for giving me the opportunity to experience the world of video production.

The Manchester Community-Technical College Respiratory Care Class of 1996, whose bright faces, keen minds, and professional spirit make me proud to be a respiratory care practitioner and a teacher.

KAM

Our students challenge us every day and, with their idealism, remind us why we chose respiratory care so many year ago ourselves. We reaffirm our commitment to the advancement and the future of the profession through them.

Our patients, who speak so eloquently to us at times of true life crisis, have been a driving force behind this project. Our mission as practitioners must always be to improve our skills so we can provide the best respiratory care to our patients and see to it that they, the most important people, are not ignored during health-care redesign, reengineering, and reform.

PFC
KAM

To the Reader/Viewer

Our goal with this comprehensive video and workbook series is to provide you with tools you can use to learn, practice, and test your clinical decision making skills. Each video addresses a separate skill area in the context of a disease or condition:

Oxygen Therapy	COPD
Aerosol Therapy	Asthma
Secretion Management	Pneumonia
Volume Expansion	Postoperative Abdominal Aortic Aneurysm
Physical Assessment	Chest Trauma
Pediatrics	Croup
Noninvasive Monitoring	Tricyclic Antidepressant Overdose
Mechanical Ventilation	Myocardial Infarction with Heart Failure and Pulmonary Edema

There are two video sets: the *Clinical Decision Series* and the *Competency Evaluation Series*. Each set has its own accompanying workbook. Videos in the *Clinical Decision Series* follow four phases of the **clinical decision-making model** through clinical case study footage and expert commentary:

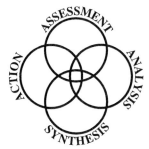 **Assessment**, in which you will collect subjective and objective data about your patient;

Analysis, in which you will review the pathophysiology relating to the assessment data;

Synthesis, where you will apply the assessment data and pathophysiology to a protocol for care; and

Action, the segment in which therapy is administered and results are evaluated

The video *Introduction to Clinical Decision Making* describes these steps in greater detail.

The *Competency Evaluation Series* provides the clinical footage alone.

THE WORKBOOK TO ACCOMPANY THE CLINICAL DECISION SERIES
The exercises in this workbook may be assigned by your instructor after you watch the video, or they may be assigned when you discuss the content areas in class. You may use this workbook as an additional resource to help you apply concepts on your own. The content and questions in this workbook can also be used as a component of your preparation for credentialling examinations.

The workbook is designed to supplement and reinforce the subject matter in each video. It is designed with a number of user-friendly features:

❑ Space is provided so that you can answer questions right in the workbook.

❑ References are provided to help you research answers.

❑ Questions are categorized by topic.

❑ Different types of questions are provided: short answer, true/false, matching, multiple choice.

❑ Follow-up questions to the video cases provide the opportunity to apply your theoretical knowledge to clinical situations.

❑ A posttest for each video topic summarizes the content to help you assess your knowledge.

❑ Answers are provided for self assessment.

❑ Sample therapist-driven protocols are in the workbook appendix.

❑ A glossary defines terms used in the videos and workbook.

The questions are designed to go beyond the content in the video and to help you apply concepts and develop critical thinking skills. You may not find the answers to all the questions in the videos themselves. Suggested references are provided to help you develop answers to questions, and a comprehensive bibliography of all source material used to develop this video and workbook series is included for your further study. These particular references are not required to answer workbook questions; any respiratory care reference text can be used. We encourage you to use other resources as well—for example, books from other disciplines such as medicine, nursing, pharmacy, and physical therapy; professionals such as RCP instructors, physicians, registered nurses, and other allied health professionals. You might decide to assemble a study group of your colleagues to discuss content, share ideas, and formulate answers.

Table of Contents

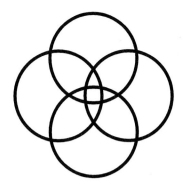

Introduction to Clinical Decision Making

Resources

Barnes TA: Core textbook of respiratory care practice, ed 2, St. Louis, 1994, Mosby.

Burton GG and Tietsort JA: Therapist-driven respiratory care protocols (TDP): a practitioner's guide, Torrance, CA, 1993, Academy Medical Systems.

Hess D: Clinical practice guidelines: why, whence, and whither? In Resp Care 40:1264-1268, 1995.

Hess D: The AARC clinical practice guidelines, Resp Care 31:1398-1401, 1991.

McCance KL and Huether SE: Pathophysiology: the biologic basis for disease in adults and children, ed 2, St. Louis, 1994, Mosby.

Price SA and Wilson LM: Pathophysiology: clinical concepts of disease processes, ed 4, St. Louis, 1992, Mosby.

Stoller JK: Why therapist-driven protocols? a balanced view, Resp Care 39:706-707, 1994.

Topic: Aspects of Clinical Decision Making

Clinical Practice Guidelines

1. What are clinical practice guidelines (CPGs)? What elements do the AARC CPGs contain?

2. Why did the American Association for Respiratory Care support the development of CPGs for respiratory care?

3. How were the AARC Clinical Practice Guidelines developed?

4. How can CPGs be used?

Therapist-Driven Protocols

5. What are therapist-driven protocols (TDPs)?

6. What are other names for TDPs?

7. Why have TDPs been developed?

8. What advantages do TDPs offer compared with traditional physician-ordered therapy?

9. What is the relationship between TDPs and the AARC Clinical Practice Guidelines?

Clinical Decision Making

10. What is the relationship between the development of clinical decision making skills and the use of TDPs?

11. Describe the four aspects of clinical decision making as presented in this series.

Pathophysiology

12. What is pathophysiology?

13. When discussing pathophysiology of the respiratory system, disorders can be divided into two major categories: obstructive patterns and restrictive patterns. Give a short definition of each, and list three disorders in each category.

14. Explain why understanding pathophysiological mechanisms will enhance the RCP's clinical decision making skills. Compare different treatments of a single symptom—dyspnea—in patients with two different pathophysiological mechanisms: (1) obstructive disease and (2) hypoxemia.

True/False

15. **T F**   Respiratory care departments throughout the country are using the AARC Clinical Practice Guidelines to develop institution-specific therapist-driven protocols and respiratory care consultation services.

16. **T F**   The AARC Clinical Practice Guidelines are the same as respiratory care protocols and critical pathways.

17. **T F**   TDPs allow for timely assessment and adjustments in a patient's respiratory care based on changes in the patient's condition.

18. **T F**   One goal of the AARC Clinical Practice Guidelines is to improve the consistency and appropriateness of respiratory care services.

19. **T F**   The use of TDPs eliminates the need for RCP-physician interaction or consultation.

20. **T F**   Pathophysiology and pathology of a disease refer to the same thing.

21. **T F**   Treatment of symptoms like cough or dyspnea will be the same, regardless of pathophysiology of the underlying disorder.

Matching

Match definition on the right to the word or phrase on the left.

22. _____ therapist-driven protocol   **A.** implementation of the care plan

23. _____ clinical practice guideline   **B.** relates pathophysiology to clinical assessment data

24. _____ synthesis   **C.** patient care plan often presented as a flow-chart

25. _____ action   **D.** includes activities like patient interview and chart review

26. _____ assessment   **E.** development of a respiratory care plan

27. _____ analysis   **F.** a set of statements defining appropriate clinical practice

                                         G. a method of universal outcome assessment

POSTTEST

1. When using the Clinical Decision-Making Model, the implementation of the respiratory care plan is part of which phase?

   a. assessment
   b. analysis
   c. synthesis
   d. action

2. The standard format of the AARC Clinical Practice Guidelines includes statements for:

   I.   assessment of need.
   II. assessment of outcome.
   III. institutional implementation.
   IV. contraindications.

       a. I and II only
       b. III and IV only
       c. I, II, and IV only
       d. all of the above

3. Development of AARC Clinical Practice Guidelines includes an extensive review process involving:

   I.   a panel of experts.
   II. consultants.
   III. AARC steering committee members.
   IV. the Agency for Health Care Policy.

       a. I and II only
       b. I, II, and III only
       c. III and IV only
       d. I, II, and IV only

4. The use of therapist- or patient-driven protocols to develop a respiratory care plan is completed in the clinical decision making phase known as:

   a. assessment.
   b. analysis.
   c. synthesis.
   d. action.

5. Physical examination of a patient to collect information as part of the decision-making process includes:

   I.   inspection.
   II. auscultation.
   III. percussion.
   IV. palpation.

       a. II only
       b. I and III only
       c. I, III, and IV only
       d. all of the above

6. When performing a thorough patient assessment as part of clinical decision making, the respiratory care practitioner will:

    I.   collect subjective data.
    II. collect objective data.
    III. review the patient's chart.
    IV. conduct a chest physical examination.

      a. I and II only
      b. III and IV only
      c. I, II, and III only
      d. all of the above

7. When you can answer this question—"What is the patient's status, and what factors in the patient's history are contributing to his or her current condition?"—you most likely have completed the phase of clinical decision making known as:

      a. assessment.
      b. analysis.
      c. synthesis.
      d. action.

8. AARC Clinical Practice Guidelines should do all of the following *except*:

      a. improve the consistency and appropriateness of care.
      b. replace institutional protocols or critical pathways.
      c. serve as a guide for education and research in the field.
      d. define and justify clinical practice.

9. Which of the following statements is/are true concerning clinical decision making?

    I.   Strong clinical decision making skills are essential to implementing TDPs.
    II. The four phases of clinical decision making should be done separately and in sequence.
    III. The ability to make clinical decisions cannot be taught; it simply develops with clinical experience.
    IV. All the information you need to make a decision about the respiratory care a patient should receive can be found in that patient's chart.

      a. I only
      b. I and II only
      c. II and III only
      d. III only

10. TDPs are respiratory care plans that:

    I.   are designed with the input of physicians.
    II. have received approval from the medical staff.
    III. have received approval from the hospital's governing body.
    IV. put the patient at the focus of attention.

      a. II and IV only
      b. I, III, and IV only
      c. I, II, and IV only
      d. all of the above

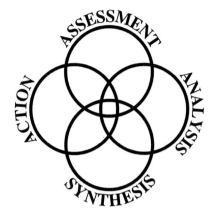

ASSESSMENT

ANALYSIS

SYNTHESIS

ACTION

Part I

Clinical Decision Series
Questions: Units 1-8

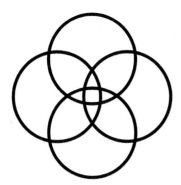

Oxygen Therapy

Resources

American Association for Respiratory Care: Clinical practice guideline: oxygen therapy in the acute care hospital, Resp Care 36:1410-1413, 1991.

American Association for Respiratory Care: Clinical practice guideline: oxygen therapy in the home or extended care facility, Resp Care 37:918-922, 1992.

American Association for Respiratory Care: Clinical practice guideline: pulse oximetry, Resp Care 36:1406-1409, 1991.

Barnes TA: Core textbook of respiratory care practice, ed 2, St. Louis, 1994, Mosby.

Scanlan CL, Spearman CB, and Sheldon RL, editors: Egan's fundamentals of respiratory care, ed 6, St. Louis, 1995, Mosby.

Shapiro BA: Clinical application of blood gases, ed 5, St. Louis, 1994, Mosby.

Wilkins RL, Krider SJ, and Sheldon RL, editors: Clinical assessment in respiratory care, ed 3, St. Louis, 1995, Mosby.

Topic 1: Oxygenation

1. State the critical values used to differentiate between mild, moderate, and severe hypoxemia in the adult patient who is less than 60 years of age.

2. Explain why a PaO_2 of less than 40 mm Hg is classified as severe hypoxemia and is a direct threat to tissue oxygenation.

3. Define the terms *uncorrected hypoxemia, corrected hypoxemia,* and *excessively corrected hypoxemia.* Include the PaO_2 values in your answer.

4. What effect does age have on the PaO_2?

5. What is cyanosis, and is it a reliable indicator of hypoxemia?

6. What is refractory hypoxemia?

7. How is oxygen carried in the blood?

8. Discuss the four physiologic causes of hypoxemia.

9. List the factors that shift the oxygen dissociation curve to the right and to the left.

        RIGHT   LEFT

10. What effect does shifting the oxygen dissociation curve to the right and to the left have on unloading oxygen at the tissues?

11. Using the oxygen dissociation curve provided below, determine the value of SaO_2 at PO_2s of 30 mm Hg, 60 mm Hg, and 90 mm Hg respectively. What can you say about the relationship between the SaO_2s and PO_2s?

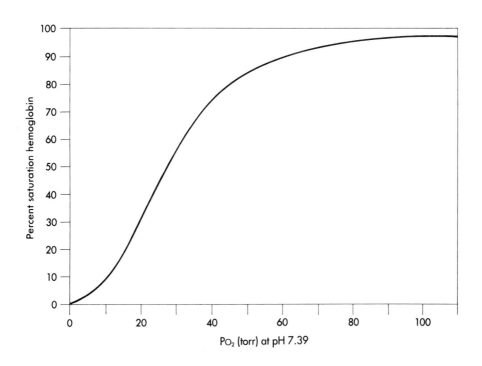

Figure 1-1   From Lane EE and Walker JF: Clinical arterial blood gas analysis, St. Louis, 1987, Mosby.

12. Differentiate between oxygen capacity and oxygen content.

13. Calculate the oxygen capacity for two patients and discuss the results. Patient A has an Hb of 16 gm/dL, SaO_2 of 95%, and a PaO_2 of 90 mm Hg. Patient B has an Hb of 8 gm/dL, SaO_2 of 95%, and a PaO_2 of 90 mm Hg.

14. Oxygen delivery to the tissues is dependent on a number of factors. List three.

15. List five deadspace-producing diseases or disorders.

16. List five shunt-producing diseases or disorders.

17. Discuss the compensatory mechanisms developed in persons with *chronic* hypoxemia.

18. Discuss the compensatory mechanisms developed in persons with *acute* hypoxemia.

19. What are the clinical signs and symptoms of hypoxemia?

20. Discuss the factors that determine delivery of oxygen to the tissues.

21. Discuss the concept of the *hypoxic drive* as it relates to oxygen therapy.

22. Each of these pictures illustrates a different aspect of $\dot{V}/\dot{Q}$ matching. Name each one, and write a brief definition of each.

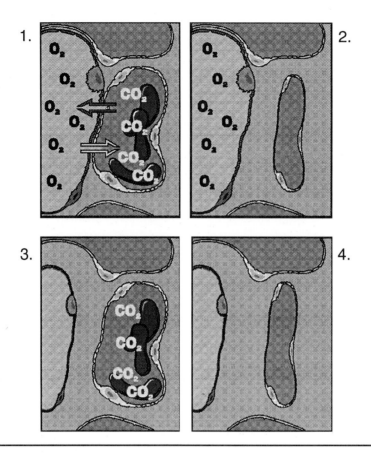

Figure 1-2 $\dot{V}/\dot{Q}$ Matching

True/False

23. **T   F**   A shift of the oxygen dissociation curve to the left results in higher SaO_2 values at the same PaO_2.

24. **T   F**   The most important compensatory mechanism for hypoxemia is increasing the cardiac output.

25. **T   F**   Normal arterial blood oxygen content is 16 to 20 ml/dL.

26. **T   F**   The oxygen dissociation curve demonstrates the linear relationship between PaO_2 and SaO_2.

27. **T   F**   It is possible for the PaO_2 and percent SaO_2 to remain unchanged while oxygen content varies with the hemoglobin level.

28. **T   F** PaO_2 is the best value with which to determine tissue oxygenation.

29. **T   F** PaO_2 reflects the ability of the lungs to allow the transfer of oxygen from the environment to the circulating blood.

30. **T   F**   The largest portion of oxygen is transported as a dissolved gas in the blood plasma.

31. **T   F** $\dot{V}/\dot{Q}$ mismatching is the most common cause of hypoxemia.

32. **T   F**   *Deadspace ventilation* is defined as "ventilation without perfusion."

33. **T   F**   Arterial oxygen content is the amount of oxygen (1) bound to hemoglobin and (2) dissolved in the plasma of arterial blood.

34. **T   F**   The most important factor indicating the oxygenation status of the arterial blood is the oxygen content.

35. **T   F**   Assessment of sensorium, vital signs, extremity temperature, and mixed venous oxygen is important to the evaluation of circulation and tissue oxygenation.

36. **T   F**   Tissue hypoxia is easily determined by measurement of PaO_2.

37. **T   F**   One gram of hemoglobin is capable of carrying 2.2 ml oxygen.

▇▇ Topic 2: Oxygen Delivery ▇▇▇▇▇▇▇▇▇▇▇▇▇▇▇▇▇▇

38. What is the overall goal when providing oxygen therapy?

39. What is meant by the term *titration* as it relates to oxygen administration?

40. Differentiate between a variable-performance device and a fixed-performance device.

41. Identify the oxygen devices pictured below and determine if the device is a fixed-performance or variable-performance device.

    A

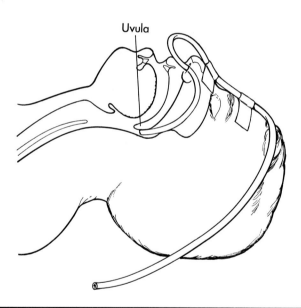

Figure 1-3a From Scanlan CL, Spearman CB, and Sheldon RL, editors: Egan's fundamentals of respiratory care, ed 6, St. Louis, 1995, Mosby.

B

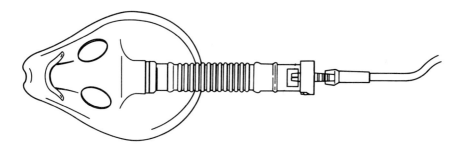

Figure 1-3b   From Kacmarek RM: In-hospital O$_2$ therapy. In Kacmarek RM, Stoller J, editors: Current respiratory care, Toronto, 1988, BC Decker.

C

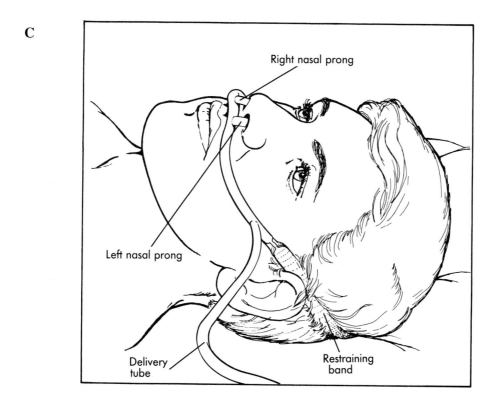

Figure 1-3c   From Scanlan CL, Spearman CB, and Sheldon RL, editors: Egan's fundamentals of respiratory care, ed 6, St. Louis, 1995, Mosby.

D

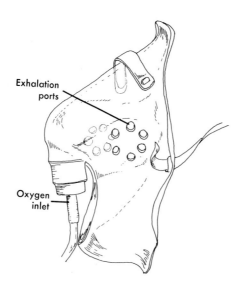

Figure 1-3d From McPherson SP: Respiratory care equipment, ed 5, St. Louis,1995, Mosby.

E

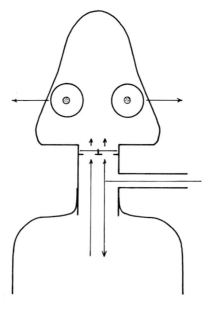

Figure 1-3e From Scanlan CL, Spearman CB, and Sheldon RL, editors: Egan's fundamentals of respiratory care, ed 6, St. Louis, 1995, Mosby.

42. List the advantages and disadvantages of the nasal cannula as an oxygen delivery device.

43. Calculate the total flow for a 35% air-entrainment mask running at 10 L/min. Does this device have enough total flow to meet the average patient's inspiratory demand?

44. You are caring for a patient admitted from the emergency department because of an exacerbation of longstanding COPD. Her respiratory rate is high, and the pattern is variable. Discuss the advantages an air-entrainment mask offers as compared with a nasal cannula in this acute situation.

45. What are the disadvantages of oxygen delivery by masks?

46. Describe how to set up a partial rebreather mask.

47. What are the advantages and disadvantages of reservoir masks for oxygen therapy?

48. What are the harmful effects of excessive oxygen?

49. List five factors that hasten the onset or increase the severity of oxygen toxicity.

50. Describe the clinical picture seen in patients exposed to high oxygen concentrations.

51. What level of oxygen is considered safe?

52. According to the AARC Clinical Practice Guidelines, what are the indications for oxygen therapy in the home?

True/False

53. **T F** During normal quiet breathing, a patient's peak inspiratory flow seldom exceeds 30 L/min but can easily double or triple in acutely ill patients.

54. **T F** When administering oxygen, it is important to always give the minimal dose needed to obtain the desired result.

55. **T F** Oxygen is indicated in adults, children, and infants older than 28 days when PaO_2 is less than 60 mm Hg or SaO_2 is less than 90% when breathing room air.

56. **T F** Partial rebreathing masks can be set up on oxygen flows of 1 to 10 L/min.

57. **T F** High-flow systems deliver a prescribed gas mixture at flowrates that exceed patient demand.

58. **T F** Air-entrainment masks set to deliver 50% oxygen or greater will easily deliver flowrates adequate to meet the inspiratory flowrates of adults in respiratory distress.

59. **T F** All oxygen delivery devices should be checked at least once per day.

60. **T F** Simple masks provide oxygen concentrations of 50% to 60% at flowrates from 5 to 10 L/min.

61. **T F** Before insertion of a nasal catheter, the distal tip should be lubricated with a water-soluble jelly.

62. **T F** The harmful effects of oxygen are determined by the PAO_2 and exposure time.

63. **T F** FIO_2s above 30% are believed to present a significant risk of absorption atelectasis.

64. **T F** PaO_2s should be kept below 80 mm Hg with low birth-weight and premature infants to minimize the risk of retinopathy of prematurity.

65. **T F** Ciliary clearance rates are increased significantly when cilia are exposed to 100% oxygen.

66. **T F** In the end stages of oxygen toxicity, hyaline membranes form in the alveolar region, and pulmonary fibrosis and hypertension develop.

67. **T F** Oxygen's toxic effect on the lung is due to the underproduction of oxygen-free radicals and loss of surfactant.

Matching

Match the oxygen device on the left to the appropriate oxygen concentration delivered on the right, based on a normal, average inspiratory flow.

68. _____ simple oxygen mask   **A.** 24%, 35%, 40%

69. _____ nasal cannula   **B.** 24%–44%

70. _____ air-entrainment mask   **C.** 21%–50%

71. _____ partial rebreathing mask **D.** 35%–50%

72. _____ nonrebreathing mask   **E.** 30%–70%

                                       F. 35%–60%

                                       G. 95%–100%

                                       H. 57%–70%

▨ Topic 3: Analysis of Oxygenation ▨

73. Explain the basic principle of operation for the pulse oximeter.

74. Discuss the documented limitations of pulse oximeters known to affect accuracy.

75. Explain how carboxyhemoglobin affects the accuracy of the pulse oximetry reading.

76. According to the AARC Clinical Practice Guidelines for pulse oximetry, what are the indications for its use?

77. According to the AARC Clinical Practice Guidelines for pulse oximetry, what are the relative contraindications for pulse oximetry measurement?

78. Describe how you would validate pulse oximeter readings.

79. When recording SpO_2 results in a patient's medical record, what information would you include?

True/False

80. **T F** Pulse oximetry is a valuable replacement for arterial blood gas measurement in critically ill patients.

81. **T F** The most reliable determination of SaO_2 is made with a cooximeter.

82. **T F** The presence of an ongoing need for measurements of pH, $PaCO_2$, total hemoglobin, and abnormal hemoglobins is a relative contraindication to pulse oximetry.

83. **T F** High/low alarms should be used with continuous and prolonged monitoring of SpO_2 .

84. **T F** Pulse oximetry is better able to accurately determine saturations below 85% than saturations above 85%.

▰ Topic 4: Follow-up to Mr. Feder ▰▰▰▰▰▰▰▰▰▰▰▰▰▰▰

Refer to the therapist-driven protocol on page 205 to complete the following.

85. You are the respiratory care practitioner who initiated the oxygen therapy for Mr. Feder. Explain the guidelines for monitoring oxygen therapy as outlined by the AARC with specific reference to their application to Mr. Feder.

86. You are the respiratory care practitioner taking care of Mr. Feder 24 hours after oxygen therapy was started. Discuss what you would evaluate to determine whether the oxygen therapy should be continued, modified, or discontinued.

87. You see Mr. Feder on the second day since oxygen therapy was initiated. His blood pressure, respiratory rate, heart rate, and temperature are all back within normal limits, and he is using a nasal cannula at 3 L/min. When you check his SpO_2, the reading on 3 L/min is 97%. What action would you take?

88. Mr. Feder has a respiratory rate of 35 to 40 breaths per minute; he is tachycardic and hypertensive. You are titrating the oxygen using a high flow device but are unable to raise his SpO_2 over 89%. What action would you take and why?

89. How does the protocol for oxygen therapy published on page 205 accommodate patients with cardiac complications? What is the physiologic basis for these accommodations?

90. Mr. Feder has been hospitalized for four days and still requires oxygen at 2 L/min. His physician requests that you evaluate him for home oxygen. How is an assessment of need performed?

91. Your initial assessment reveals a patient admitted for viral pneumonia with a history of bronchitis, and open-heart surgery five years ago. His respiratory rate is 32, heart rate 108, BP 145/95, and the SpO_2 is 86%. He is extremely restless. What action should you take?

POSTTEST

1. Regardless of age, any adult patient with a PaO_2 of less than _____ mm Hg indicates severe hypoxemia.

    a. 20
    b. 40
    c. 60
    d. 80

2. Arterial hypoxemia in adults is defined as a PaO_2 less than _____ mm Hg when breathing room air.

    a. 100
    b. 90
    c. 80
    d. 70

3. Studies have shown the typical disposable nonrebreathing mask delivers an FIO_2 between:

    a. .57 and .70
    b. .35 and .60
    c. .90 and 1.00
    d. .24 and .44

4. Two major categories of high-flow devices include:

    a. reservoir and backfill systems.
    b. air-entrainment and blending systems.
    c. blending and reservoir systems.
    d. variable performance and air-entrainment systems.

5. Which of the following have been shown to affect readings, limit precision, or limit the performance of a pulse oximeter?

    I.   hyperbilirubinemia
    II. motion artifact
    III. low perfusion states
    IV. intravascular dyes

        a. IV only
        b. I and III only
        c. II, III, and IV only
        d. all of the above

6. The oxygen dissociation curve is shifted to the left by:

    I.   carboxyhemoglobin
    II. decreased body temperature
    III. alkalosis
    IV. increased $PaCO_2$

        a. I and II only
        b. III and IV only
        c. I, II, and III only
        d. all of the above

7. As a general rule of thumb, a total output flow of at least _____ L/min is needed for high-flow devices to meet or exceed patients' inspiratory demands.

   a. 60
   b. 10
   c. 30
   d. 75

8. Which of the following patients is most likely to develop oxygen toxicity?

   a. a patient on FIO_2 of 0.4 with a PaO_2 of 70 mm Hg
   b. a patient on FIO_2 of 0.6 with a PaO_2 of 55 mm Hg
   c. a patient on FIO_2 of 0.4 with a PaO_2 of 95 mm Hg
   d. a patient on FIO_2 of 0.9 with a PaO_2 of 122 mm Hg

9. Patients who stop breathing from a loss of their hypoxic drive mechanism do so because of an increased:

   a. PaO_2.
   b. PAO_2.
   c. FIO_2.
   d. Hb.

10. Indications for oxygen therapy in the acute care hospital include documented hypoxemia (in subjects breathing room air), defined as:

    a. $PaO_2 \leq 55$ mm Hg or $SaO_2 \leq 88\%$.
    b. $PaO_2 \leq 60$ mm Hg or $SaO_2 \leq 90\%$.
    c. $PaO_2 \leq 80$ mm Hg or $SaO_2 \leq 92\%$.
    d. none of the above

11. Carbon monoxide poisoning is an example of which type of hypoxemia?

    a. histotoxic
    b. circulatory
    c. hypoxic
    d. anemic

12. According to the AARC Clinical Practice Guidelines for oxygen therapy in the acute care hospital, once oxygen therapy is initiated, the patient should be monitored, including measurement of oxygen tensions or saturation within:

    I.   12 hours of initiation with FIO_2 less than 0.40.
    II. 8 hours with FIO_2 greater than 0.40 (including postanesthesia recovery).
    III. 72 hours in acute myocardial infarction.
    IV. 2 hours for any patient with the principal diagnosis of COPD.

       a. I and II only
       b. III and IV only
       c. II, III, and IV only
       d. all of the above

13. Which of the following are true concerning the nasal cannula?

   I.   The FIO_2 depends on the patient's rate and depth of breathing.
   II. With liter flows greater than 4 L/min, it is a fixed-performance device.
   III. Flows above 6 to 8 L/min can cause nasal dryness and bleeding.
   IV. Use should be limited to patients with a stable respiratory rate and pattern.

   a. I and III only
   b. I, III, and IV only
   c. II and IV only
   d. all of the above

14. Absorption atelectasis is a concern as the _____ increases.

   a. FIO_2
   b. PaO_2
   c. CaO_2
   d. $\dot{V}/\dot{Q}$

15. The lowest acceptable PaO_2 for a 70-year-old patient is about:

   a. 70 mm Hg.
   b. 60 mm Hg.
   c. 65 mm Hg.
   d. 75 mm Hg.

16. When a patient has a hemoglobin level of 11 gm%, cyanosis will most likely appear when _____ gm% hemoglobin is saturated with oxygen.

   a. 5
   b. 6
   c. 8
   d. 9

17. Which of the following are true concerning air-entrainment masks?

   I.   They are best used for short periods when precise FIO_2s are needed.
   II. They can ensure stable FIO_2s to most patients who require less than 35% oxygen.
   III. They deliver a stable FIO_2 in all concentrations, including 60% and higher.
   IV. Because of size, discomfort, and appearance, they are less well-tolerated over time as compared with nasal cannulas.

   a. I and III only
   b. I, II, and IV only
   c. II, III, and IV only
   d. all of the above

18. Which of the following results, when the patient is breathing room air, indicates the need for home oxygen?

   a. $PaO_2 \leq 55$ mm Hg or $SaO_2 \leq 88\%$
   b. $PaO_2 \leq 60$ mm Hg or $SaO_2 \leq 90\%$
   c. $PaO_2 \leq 59$ mm Hg or $SaO_2 \leq 89\%$
   d. $PaO_2 \leq 80$ mm Hg or $SaO_2 \leq 92\%$

19. Harmful effects of excessive oxygen include:

    I.   altered surfactant production.
    II. oxygen-induced hypoventilation.
    III. depression of ciliary activity.
    IV. retinopathy of prematurity.

        a. I and III only
        b. II only
        c. III only
        d. all of the above

20. Oxygen saturation is best defined as:

    a. the total amount of oxygen dissolved in the plasma, expressed as a percentage of the total.
    b. an index of the actual amount of oxygen bound to hemoglobin, expressed as a percentage of the total capacity.
    c. the amount of oxygen dissolved in the plasma plus the amount bound to hemoglobin.
    d. a measurement of the tension of oxygen.

21. The most common cause of hypoxemia in patients with respiratory dysfunction is:

    a. $\dot{V}/\dot{Q}$ mismatching.
    b. hypoventilation.
    c. diffusion defect.
    d. anemia.

22. Common clinical manifestations of hypoxemia include:

    I.   confusion.
    II. tachycardia.
    III. tachypnea.
    IV. hypotension.

        a. I and III only
        b. I, II, and III only
        c. II, III, and IV only
        d. all of the above

23. The major difference between the partial rebreathing mask and the nonrebreathing mask is the:

    a. size of the reservoir bag.
    b. the liter flow that is set to keep the bag from deflating.
    c. the one-way valve between the mask and reservoir.
    d. the design of the face mask.

24. Extreme degrees of $\dot{V}/\dot{Q}$ mismatching include:

    I.   deadspace ventilation.
    II. shunt.
    III. diffusion defect.
    IV. hypoventilation.

       a. I and II only
       b. III and IV only
       c. II, III, and IV only
       d. all of the above

25. A shunt greater than _____ % results in hypoxemia.

    a. 5
    b. 10
    c. 12
    d. 15

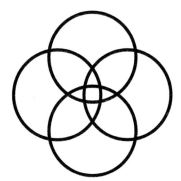

Aerosol Therapy

Resources

American Association for Respiratory Care: Clinical practice guideline: bland aerosol administration, Resp Care 38:1196-1200, 1993.

American Association for Respiratory Care: Clinical practice guideline: selection of aerosol delivery device, Resp Care 37:891-897, 1992.

Barnes TA: Core textbook of respiratory care practice, ed 2, St. Louis, 1994, Mosby.

McPherson SP: Respiratory care equipment, ed 5, St. Louis, 1995, Mosby.

Scanlan CL, Spearman CB, and Sheldon RL, editors: Egan's fundamentals of respiratory care, ed 6, St. Louis, 1995, Mosby.

Topic 1: Aerosol Therapy Equipment

1. Define *aerosol*.

2. List four of the six factors that affect the deposition of aerosol particles.

3. What is MMAD?

4. What is the optimal size for aerosol particles to be delivered to the lungs?

5. Describe a metered dose inhaler (MDI).

6. How can you estimate the amount of medication remaining in an MDI canister?

7. Describe the advantages of dry powder inhalers (DPIs).

8. What are the disadvantages of DPIs?

9. Describe two techniques used to minimize drug loss during small-volume nebulizer therapy.

10. Describe the optimal placement of the small-volume nebulizer for patients receiving treatments while on mechanical ventilation.

11. Describe the advantages of using large-volume nebulizers to administer bronchodilators and other medications to the lung.

12. Discuss why patients must be monitored closely for drug toxicity during continuous nebulization therapy.

13. What are the indications for medicated aerosol therapy?

14. Describe the hazards/complications of medicated aerosol therapy.

15. Describe the limitations of MDI therapy.

16. Describe the limitations of DPIs.

17. Describe the limitations of small-volume nebulizer therapy.

18. Describe the limitations of ultrasonic nebulization therapy.

19. Explain why MDI with spacer is often the preferred method of administration of aerosol delivery to the airways.

20. What should a respiratory care practitioner monitor while administering aerosol therapy to a patient?

21. Describe the infection control procedures that should be employed with aerosol delivery.

22. Discuss the criteria that support the choice of the small-volume nebulizer over the other delivery techniques.

23. Discuss the basic principle of operation for the ultrasonic nebulizer.

24. What is the name of the device manufactured specifically for the administration of ribavirin and how does this device differ from most nebulizers?

25. Describe the basic principle of operation of the Babbington nebulizer.

True/False

26. **T F** Jet nebulizers use the Bernoulli principle to draw water up a capillary tube and a baffle to reduce the aerosol particle size.

27. **T F** A ball placed in the path of the aerosol, the surface of the water in a container, or the sides of the container can all serve as baffles.

28. **T F** The main distinguishing feature of the sidestream nebulizer is the fact that the main flow of gas passes through the aerosol generator.

29. **T F** Use of a spacer with an MDI for administration of steroid medications is recommended to ensure proper dosing and reduce particle impact in the mouth.

30. **T F** Aerosols with an MMAD of 0.8 to 2.0 microns are targeted to the lung parenchyma, whereas particles less than 0.8 microns are often exhaled.

31. **T F**   Aerosol delivery to the lungs is dependent on the size of the particles, inhalation technique, and airway caliber.

32. **T F**   Slow inspiratory flows are associated with greater deposition of drug within the upper airway due to impaction.

33. **T F**   The decreased size of airways associated with bronchospasm restricts the flow of aerosol to targeted distal airways.

34. **T F**   High inspiratory flow rates result in greater distribution of aerosol to the larger airways and nongravity-dependent areas of the lung as compared with slower inspiratory flow rates.

35. **T F**   Drug delivery by aerosol has a high therapeutic index because the method delivers a high drug concentration to the airway directly, with very low systemic dosing, thereby minimizing systemic side effects.

36. **T F**   The performance of small-volume nebulizers is not affected by factors such as humidity and temperature.

37. **T F**   Tachypnea is associated with a decreased opportunity for medication deposition because there is less time for the drug to settle out of suspension.

38. **T F**   A number of studies have demonstrated that the dose of the drug delivered per puff by MDI is greater when administered to ventilated patients as compared with spontaneously breathing patients.

39. **T F**   The MMAD of most MDIs is between 3 and 6 microns with a deposition in the lung of about 50%.

40. **T F**   The autohaler (3M) is an example of a device developed to allow for flow-triggered actuation of the MDI in an effort to eliminate the need for hand-breath coordination.

Matching

Match the equipment pictured on the following pages (Figures 2-1a to 2-1g) with the proper descriptor below.

41. _____   Babbington nebulizer

42. _____   dry powder inhaler

43. _____   ultrasonic nebulizer

44. _____   large-volume nebulizer

45. _____   MDI with spacer

46. _____   small-volume nebulizer

47. _____   small particle aerosol generator

A

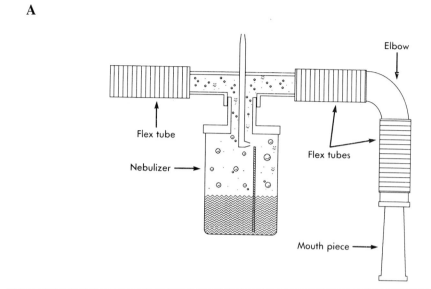

Figure 2-1a From McPherson SP: Respiratory care equipment, ed 5, St. Louis,1995, Mosby.

B

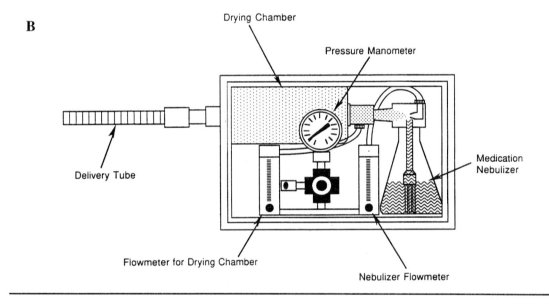

Figure 2-1b From McPherson SP: Respiratory care equipment, ed 5, St. Louis,1995, Mosby.

C

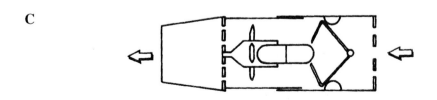

Figure 2-1c From Scanlan CL, Spearman CB, and Sheldon RL, editors: Egan's fundamentals of respiratory care, ed 6, St. Louis, 1995, Mosby.

D

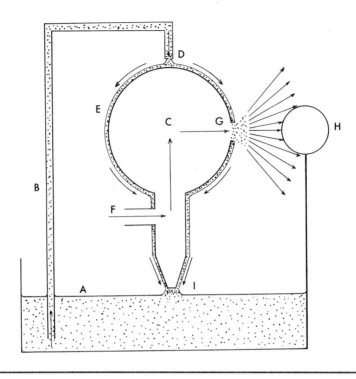

Figure 2-1d From Scanlan CL, Spearman CB, and Sheldon RL, editors: Egan's fundamentals of respiratory care, ed 6, St. Louis, 1995, Mosby.

E

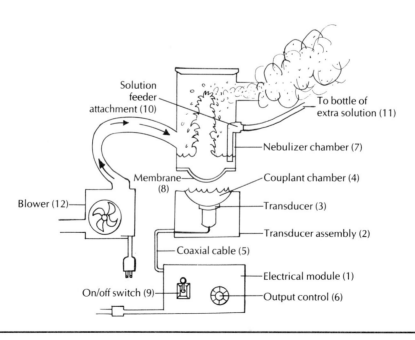

Figure 2-1e From Scanlan CL, Spearman CB, and Sheldon RL, editors: Egan's fundamentals of respiratory care, ed 6, St. Louis, 1995, Mosby.

F

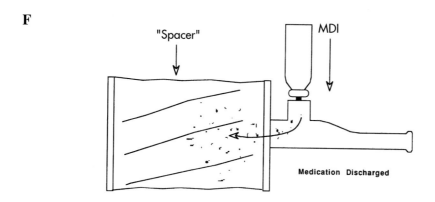

Figure 2-1f From McPherson SP: Respiratory care equipment, ed 5, St. Louis,1995, Mosby.

G

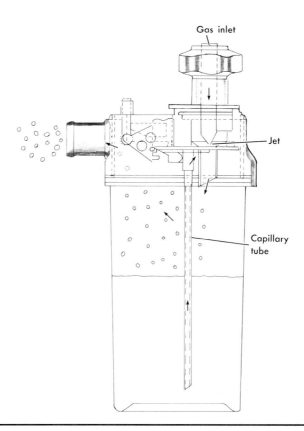

Figure 2-1g From McPherson SP: Respiratory care equipment, ed 5, St. Louis,1995, Mosby.

▬ Topic 2: Bland Aerosol Administration ▬▬▬▬▬▬▬▬

48. What is bland aerosol therapy?

49. List the indications for bland aerosol administration.

50. What are the contraindications for bland aerosol administration?

51. List the hazards and/or complications of bland aerosol administration.

52. Discuss what you would monitor while administering a bland aerosol treatment to a patient.

True/False

53. **T F** Large-volume nebulizers, ultrasonic nebulizers, mist tents, and Babbington nebulizers can be used for bland aerosol administration.

54. **T F** Aerosol therapy with bland solutions is used for diagnostic purposes only.

55. **T F** One problem encountered with the use of large-volume nebulizers at high flow rates is excessive noise.

56. **T F** High-density bland aerosol production by ultrasonic nebulization and less dense aerosolization of water can cause reactive bronchospasm and increased airway resistance in some patients.

57. **T F** Respiratory care practitioners must ensure that patients are capable of clearing secretions once they are mobilized by bland aerosol therapy.

58. **T F** A hazard of continuous nebulization of sterile fluid is overhydration in select patient populations.

59. **T F** Excessive nebulization of normal saline has the potential to cause a fluid and electrolyte imbalance, such as hypernatremia.

60. **T F** To date, there are no published reports of nosocomial infection due to *Legionella pneumophila.*

61. **T F** The organism most commonly associated with the contamination of aerosol generators is *Pseudomonas aeruginosa.*

62. **T F** Stridor, hoarseness following extubation, and discomfort associated with airway instrumentation or insult are all indications for the administration of bland aerosols.

Topic 3: Follow-up to Mr. Carr

Refer to the therapist-driven protocol on page 206 to complete the following.

63. What factors must the respiratory care practitioner consider when determining how aerosolized medication is to be delivered to the patient?

64. During the initial visit with Mr. Carr, it was observed that he was extremely anxious, with a respiratory rate of 40 to 45 breaths per minute. Would he be a candidate for MDI or small-volume nebulization of the bronchodilator?

65. Mr. Carr is treated for his exacerbation of asthma for 24 hours by small-volume nebulization with Proventil (albuterol) every 4 hours. You notice he is calmer and that he has a respiratory rate of 18, heart rate of 70, and scattered expiratory wheezes on auscultation. Would you recommend any changes in the delivery of the therapy at this time?

66. You are evaluating Mr. Carr's technique with his MDI and spacer, and you notice he exhales immediately after actuation of the dose. Is this a problem, considering that he is using a spacer?

67. You are treating Mr. Carr on the second day of his admission. His pretreatment peak flow was 350 L/min, and his posttreatment peak flow was 460 L/min. Should his therapy be continued?

68. During the second day of Mr. Carr's admission, his peak flows have returned to his green zone, breath sounds denote good aeration with a few scattered expiratory wheezes, and he appears to be much calmer. He has received all of his treatments by small-volume nebulizer. Should his therapy continue unchanged? If you think it should change, explain the recommendations you would make.

69. Explain what you would include when instructing a patient on the proper technique for use of an MDI without a spacer.

1. Limitations of the MDI include all of the following *except*:

    a. environmental concerns (chlorofluorocarbons).
    b. clumping, as a possible result of humidity.
    c. improper technique.
    d. inadequate instruction.

2. Holding chambers differ from spacers in that they:

    a. reduce oropharyngeal deposition of the medication.
    b. reduce the need for hand-breath coordination.
    c. prevent remaining aerosol from being cleared with exhalation.
    d. do not use a mask assembly.

3. Aerosol particles in the 2- to 5-micron range will most likely be deposited in the:

    a. upper airways.
    b. bronchi.
    c. alveoli.
    d. bronchioles.

4. Ultrasonic nebulizers determine the particle size of the aerosol produced by the:

    a. set frequency.
    b. amplitude adjustment.
    c. baffle series.
    d. shearing forces created.

5. Holding chamber accessory devices used with MDIs are beneficial because they:

    I.   eliminate the need for hand-breath coordination.
    II. eliminate the need to rinse the mouth after corticosteroid use.
    III. improve the delivery of medication to the lower airway.
    IV. reduce oropharyngeal deposition.

        a. IV only
        b. I and III only
        c. I, III, and IV only
        d. all of the above

6. Potential hazards/complications of aerosol delivery devices include which of the following?

    I.   cardiotoxic effects of Freon with excessive use of the MDI
    II. underdosing due to malfunction and/or improper technique
    III. overdosing due to malfunction and/or improper technique
    IV. stimulation of the parasympathetic nervous system

        a. I and II only
        b. III and IV only
        c. I, II, and III only
        d. all of the above

7. Nebulizers incorporate baffles to:

   a. ensure one-way flow of aerosol particles.
   b. reduce aerosol particle size.
   c. increase nebulizer output.
   d. mix solutions.

8. Drugs targeted for the lung parenchyma should have a particle size of:

   a. 5 to 10 microns.
   b. 2 to 5 microns.
   c. 1 to 2 microns.
   d. less than 1 micron.

9. To maximize the aerosol deposition with an MDI, the user should:

   I.   take slow deep breaths with administration.
   II. hold his or her breath at end inspiration for 10 seconds.
   III. activate the MDI before beginning inspiration.
   IV. take rapid, deep breaths with administration.

   a. I and II only
   b. II, III, and IV only
   c. I, II, and IV only
   d. all of the above

10. According to the AARC Clinical Practice Guideline for selection of an aerosol delivery device, limitations of the ultrasonic nebulizer include:

    I.   the cost of the device.
    II. its mechanical reliability.
    III. its vulnerability to contamination.
    IV. the need for an electrical power source.

    a. II and IV only
    b. I, III, and IV only
    c. I, II, and IV only
    d. all of the above

11. Which device is best suited to provide aerosol delivery to the lower airways?

    a. nebulizer A—MMAD of 50 to 80 microns
    b. nebulizer B—MMAD of 2 to 5 microns
    c. nebulizer C—MMAD of 0.5 to 2 microns
    d. nebulizer D—MMAD of 5 to 10 microns

12. Factors that affect aerosol deposition include:

   I.   patient ventilatory pattern.
   II. aerosol particle size.
   III. airway anatomy and caliber.
   IV. inspiratory flow rate.

      a. I and II only
      b. III and IV only
      c. II, III, and IV only
      d. all of the above

13. Drugs available in DPI form in the United States include:

   I.   cromolyn sodium.
   II. albuterol.
   III. Proventil.
   IV. acetylcysteine.

      a. I and II only
      b. I and IV only
      c. III and IV only
      d. I, II, and IV only

14. A breath hold of _____ seconds has been reported to provide optimal aerosol deposition with MDI use.

   a. 3
   b. 5
   c. 7
   d. 10

15. High inspiratory flow rates are associated with greater deposition of aerosolized drug within the upper airways due to:

   a. gravitational sedimentation.
   b. inertial impaction.
   c. Brownian movement.
   d. diffusion.

16. Advantages of DPIs include which of the following?

   I.   DPIs are relatively inexpensive.
   II. DPIs do not depend on the use of chlorofluorocarbons.
   III. DPIs do not require hand-breath coordination.
   IV. Most bronchodilators are available in this form.

      a. I and II only
      b. II and III only
      c. I, II, and III only
      d. all of the above

17. Bland aerosol therapy can be administered by which of the following devices?

    I.   ultrasonic nebulizer
    II. mist tent
    III. large-volume nebulizer
    IV. Babbington nebulizer

        a. I and III only
        b. I and II only
        c. II, III, and IV only
        d. all of the above

18. A coupling chamber is part of the:

    a. ultrasonic nebulizer.
    b. small particle aerosol generator.
    c. aerochamber.
    d. centrifugal nebulizer.

19. Drug reconcentration is a potential problem with:

    I.   multiple dosing using an MDI with a spacer.
    II. thirty minutes of ultrasonic nebulization.
    III. unsupervised small-volume nebulizer therapy.
    IV. use of DPIs in high humidity environments.

        a. II only
        b. III only
        c. I and II only
        d. all of the above

20. According to the Centers for Disease Control and Prevention, recommendations for the care of nebulization reservoir systems include:

    I.   using sterile equipment.
    II. changing or replacing with sterile water every 24 hours.
    III. using tap water only as a diluent.
    IV. restricting devices to single-patient use or subjecting them to high-level disinfection between patients.

        a. I and II only
        b. I and III only
        c. I, II, and IV only
        d. all of the above

21. Continuous nebulization of bronchodilators may be indicated when the:

    I.   patient does not respond to standard dosing.
    II. medication needs to be delivered while the patient sleeps.
    III. patient is receiving treatments every 15 minutes.
    IV. patient prefers delivery by mask.

        a. I and II only
        b. I, II, and III only
        c. III and IV only
        d. all of the above

22. Indications for bland aerosol therapy administration include:

    I.   the presence of an artificial tracheal airway.
    II. a spontaneous cough that fails to clear secretions.
    III. postoperative upper abdominal or thoracic surgery.
    IV. the presence of subglottic or postextubation edema.

        a. I and IV only
        b. I, II, and III only
        c. II, III, and IV only
        d. all of the above

23. Assessment of outcome of aerosol therapy might include:

    I.   measurement of FEV_1 or peak flow.
    II. patient response to, or compliance with, the procedure.
    III. proper technique in applying the device.

        a. I and II only
        b. II and III only
        c. I and III only
        d. all of the above

24. A patient in the emergency department has an FEV_1 of 1920 ml before bronchodilator therapy and an FEV_1 of 2300 ml after therapy. What is her percentage of improvement?

    a. 20%
    b. 23%
    c. 35%
    d. 83%

25. The most effective way to improve aerosol deposition when using a small-volume nebulizer is to:

    a. use slow inspiratory flows.
    b. add a 50-ml expiratory reservoir.
    c. take deep breaths.
    d. use a 3- to 5-second breath hold.

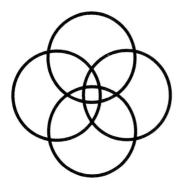

Secretion Management

Resources

American Association for Respiratory Care: Clinical practice guideline: postural drainage therapy, Resp Care 36:1418-1426, 1991.

Barnes TA: Core textbook of respiratory care practice, ed 2, St. Louis, 1994, Mosby.

Scanlan CL, Spearman CB, and Sheldon RL, editors: Egan's fundamentals of respiratory care, ed 6, St. Louis, 1995, Mosby.

Wilkins RL, Krider SJ, and Sheldon RL, editors: Clinical assessment in respiratory care, ed 3, St. Louis, 1995, Mosby.

Topic 1: Mucociliary Transport

1. Describe normal respiratory mucus clearance.

2. Identify the respiratory cilia, gel layer, and sol layer in the diagram below.

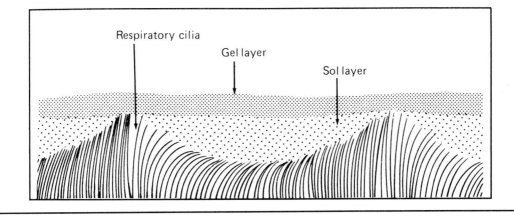

Figure 3-1   From Martin DE and Youtsey JW: Respiratory anatomy and physiology, St. Louis, 1988, Mosby.

3. List three factors that disrupt normal respiratory mucus clearance.

4. Describe how a normal cough is generated.

5. Label the four phases of a cough pictured in the diagram below.

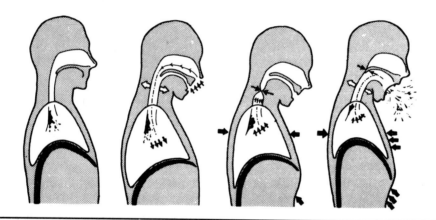

Figure 3-2   From Cherniack RM and Cherniack L: Respiration in health and disease, ed 3, Philadelphia, 1983, WB Saunders.

6. Name all of the lung segments for the right and left upper, middle, and lower lobes.

True/False

7. **T F** Endotracheal intubation can severely compromise the respiratory system's ability to warm and humidify inspired gases because it bypasses the nose.

8. **T F** In the nose, the ciliary escalator propels material back to the pharynx.

9. **T F** Drying of the respiratory mucosa inhibits ciliary activity.

10. **T F** Smoking is known to stimulate ciliary activity.

11. **T F** The nose, pharynx, and larynx conduct gases to and from the lungs and serve as the frontline defense mechanism.

▬ Topic 2: Pneumonia ▬

12. What are four common types of pneumonia seen in adults?

13. Differentiate between the following radiographic patterns: alveolar, interstitial bronchopneumonia, lobar, and necrotizing.

14. Discuss pneumococcal pneumonia, including its clinical presentation and treatment.

15. List four examples of viruses known to cause pneumonia.

16. Give five examples of conditions in which host defenses are impaired, thus predisposing that host to the development of pneumonia.

17. Describe the chest physical assessment findings that are consistent with the diagnosis of lobar pneumonia.

18. Give three examples each of unusual organisms responsible for pneumonia in the normal and the abnormal host.

19. List four organisms most commonly associated with nosocomial pneumonia.

20. Describe the difference between nosocomial colonization and nosocomial infection as it relates to the respiratory system.

Matching

Match the description of sputum on the left with the possible cause on the right.

21. _____ mucoid

A. pulmonary embolism with infarction, neoplasm, tuberculosis

22. _____ rusty

B. bronchial asthma, emphysema, early chronic bronchitis

23. _____ red currant jelly

C. smoke or coal dust inhalation

24. _____ black

D. pulmonary edema

25. _____ frothy white or pink

E. *Haemophilus influenzae* pneumonia

26. _____ foul-smelling

F. bronchiectasis, advanced chronic bronchitis

27. _____ yellow or green, copious

G. lung abscess, anaerobic infections, bronchiectasis

28. _____ mucopurulent

H. infection, pneumonia, cystic fibrosis

I. *Klebsiella pneumonia*

J. *Pneumococcal pneumonia*

K. broncholithiasis, aspiration of foreign material

True/False

29. **T F** The AIDS epidemic has increased the incidence of what were once considered to be rare pneumonias such as *Pneumocystis carinii*, *Mycobacterium avium-intracellulare*, and *cytomegalovirus*.

30. **T F** *S. pneumoniae, S. aureus, P. aeruginosa,* and *M. tuberculosis* are examples of viruses that can cause pneumonia in the adult patient.

31. **T F** Treatment of *Pneumococcal* pneumonia often involves antibiotic therapy, bed rest, pain medication, pulmonary physical therapy, adequate hydration, and oxygen therapy.

32. **T F** *Hemophilus influenzae* pneumonia is usually seen in children but can also cause pneumonia in adults.

33. **T F** Patients with *Mycoplasma* pneumonia complain of fever, myalgia, nonpleuritic chest pain, headache, and minimally productive cough.

34. **T F** Legionnaires' disease is caused by *Legionella intracellulare*.

35. **T F** Pulmonary tuberculosis is an infection caused by the acid-fast bacillus known as *Mycobacterium tuberculosis*.

36. **T F** Impaired host defenses such as those seen with AIDS, diabetes, and alcoholism predispose the host to pneumonia.

37. **T F** Mycoses are fungal infections.

38. **T F** Immunocompromised hosts are susceptible to several viral pneumonias including *cytomegalovirus*, *varicella zoster*, and *herpes simplex*.

Topic 3: Chest Physical Therapy

39. Write five goals of chest physical therapy.

40. Define the term *chest physical therapy*.

41. According to the AARC Clinical Practice Guidelines for postural drainage therapy, what are the indications for turning the patient?

42. According to the AARC Clinical Practice Guidelines for postural drainage therapy, what are the indications for postural drainage?

43. According to the AARC Clinical Practice Guidelines for postural drainage therapy, what are the indications for external manipulation of the thorax?

44. What are four *acute* conditions for which chest physical therapy is indicated?

45. What are four *chronic* conditions for which chest physical therapy is indicated?

46. What are some of the preventive uses of chest physical therapy?

47. What are the three primary objectives of therapeutic positioning?

48. Describe what should be included in the initial patient assessment done to determine the need for chest physical therapy.

49. What are the two *absolute* contraindications to postural drainage?

50. What are four *relative* contraindications to postural drainage?

51. What patient parameters should the respiratory care practitioner monitor when performing postural drainage?

52. Describe the outcome criteria indicating successful postural drainage.

53. Describe what should be included in the documentation of a chest physical therapy session including postural drainage, percussion, and vibration.

54. Describe segmental breathing exercises.

55. Describe lateral costal breathing exercises.

56. What is pursed lip breathing, and why does it help patients breathe easier?

57. What is the purpose of teaching a patient the directed cough technique?

58. List four indications for directed cough.

59. What modifications are made for surgical patients performing the directed cough maneuver?

60. Describe the forced expiration technique (also known as "huff" coughing).

61. What is PEP therapy and how does it help mobilize secretions?

62. What steps can the respiratory care practitioner take to minimize the risk of hypoxemia in patients who are at risk during chest physical therapy sessions?

63. You are performing postural drainage and percussion on a patient when she begins to vomit. According to the AARC Clinical Practice Guidelines, what action should you take?

64. You are called to start chest physical therapy on a young woman admitted with fever, malaise, and increased sputum production. She has cystic fibrosis and uses a flutter valve at home. Following her first session of postural drainage with percussion and vibration, her breath sounds reveal an increase in adventitious sounds as compared with diminished breath sounds prior to the start of therapy. Should the therapy be continued or discontinued at this point? Why?

65. Describe autogenic drainage.

66. Describe the high-frequency chest wall compression (HFCC) system.

67. What advantages does the position seen in the diagram below offer patients experiencing shortness of breath?

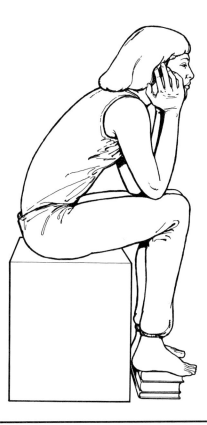

Figure 3-3 From Scanlan CL, Spearman CB, and Sheldon RL, editors: Egan's fundamentals of respiratory care, ed 6, St. Louis, 1995, Mosby.

68. Describe diaphragmatic breathing.

Matching

Match the segment that is being drained in the following diagrams (Figures 3-4a to 3-4e) to the descriptors below. Answers should be used only once.

A. both lower lobes, posterior segments

B. left lower lobe, lateral segment

C. right middle lobe

D. right upper lobe, posterior segment

E. superior segment, lower lobes

F. superior and inferior lingular segment

G. right upper lobe, apical segment

69. _____

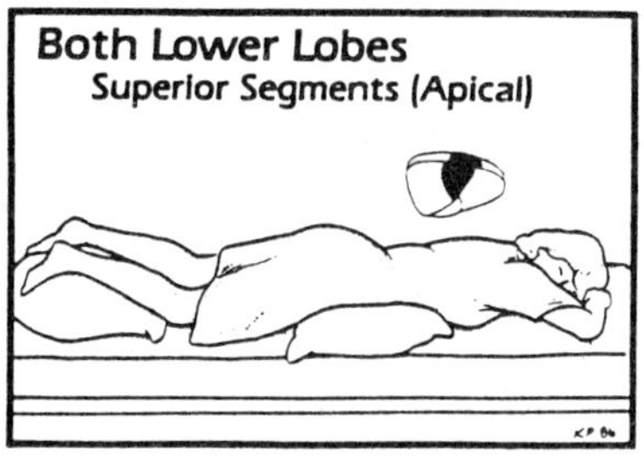

Both Lower Lobes
Superior Segments (Apical)

70. _____

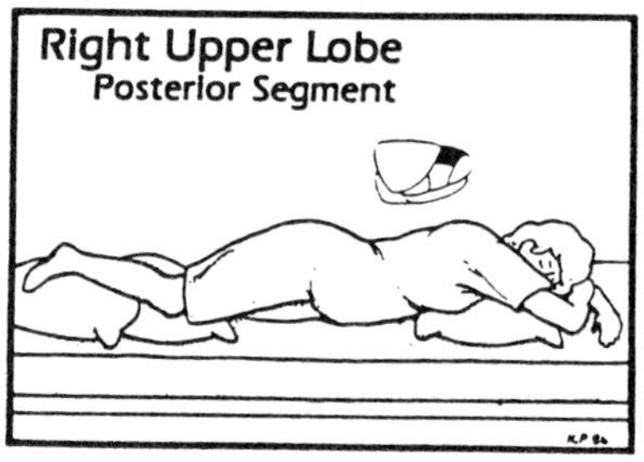

Right Upper Lobe
Posterior Segment

71. _____

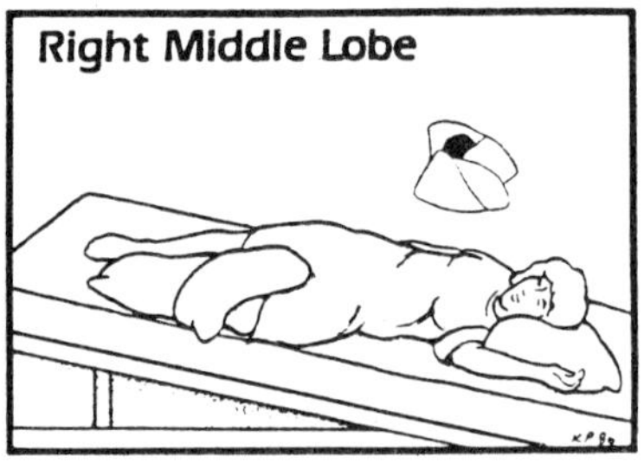

Right Middle Lobe

72. _____

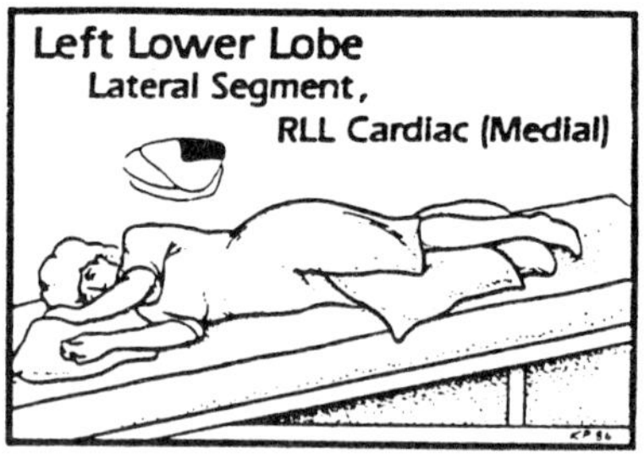

Left Lower Lobe
Lateral Segment,
RLL Cardiac (Medial)

73. _____

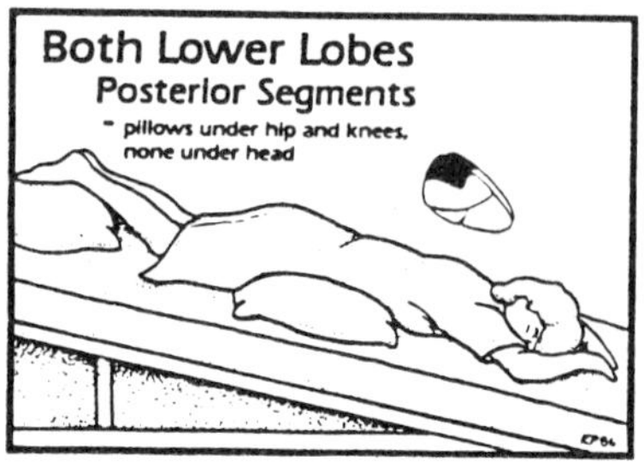

Both Lower Lobes
Posterior Segments
* pillows under hip and knees,
none under head

Figure 3-4a–e From Frownfelter DL: Chest physical therapy and pulmonary rehabilitation: an interdisciplinary approach, ed 2, St. Louis, 1987, Mosby.

True/False

74. **T F** Postural drainage treatment times should be scheduled either before or at least 1 1/2 to 2 hours after meals or tube feedings to reduce the chance of vomiting and aspiration by the patient.

75. **T F** Diseases such as cystic fibrosis, bronchiectasis, and cavitating lung disease often benefit from postural drainage.

76. **T F** Adequate systemic and airway hydration is important to the success of postural drainage therapy.

77. **T F** Postural drainage positions should be held for 3 to 15 minutes, as tolerated, and longer if good sputum production results.

78. **T F** Oxygen saturation monitoring is beneficial during postural drainage sessions since patients can desaturate during the procedure.

79. **T F** A patient's subjective response to chest physical therapy should never be included as outcome criteria.

80. **T F** The application of vibration to the chest wall is designed to jar retained secretions loose from the tracheobronchial walls.

81. **T F** Vibration is applied during the inspiratory and expiratory phases following postural drainage.

82. **T F** High-frequency chest wall compression is a mechanical technique designed to aid secretion removal.

83. **T F** Directed coughing is most effective in clearing secretions from the peripheral airways.

84. **T F** The forced expiration technique consists of forced expirations from mid-to-low lung volume without closure of the glottis, followed by a period of diaphragmatic breathing and relaxation.

85. **T F** Placing the "good lung" in the down position enhances oxygenation in patients with unilateral lung disease.

86. **T F** Changes in vital signs are to be expected during chest physical therapy sessions; bradycardia, tachycardia, and irregularities in pulse or blood pressure should be ignored.

87. **T F** The primary purpose of diaphragmatic breathing exercises is to promote greater use of the diaphragm and to decrease the use of the accessory muscles of inspiration.

Topic 4: Follow-up to Mr. Gonsalves

Refer to the therapist-driven protocol on page 207 to complete the following.

88. You are the respiratory care practitioner taking care of Mr. Gonsalves on the second day since chest physical therapy was started. Discuss what you would evaluate to determine if the therapy should be continued, modified, or discontinued.

89. You see Mr. Gonsalves on the third day of chest physical therapy. He is producing small amounts of white secretions, he is afebrile, his vital signs are normal, and his oxygen has been discontinued. When you auscultate his chest, you note that he has improved aeration in the right middle lobe and that his lungs are otherwise clear. His chest radiograph shows clearing of the consolidation. What would you recommend and why?

90. You see Mr. Gonsalves 24 hours after postural drainage and percussion was begun. He has received three sessions of postural drainage with percussion. The RCP's records state that the patient tolerates the therapy well and that he produces 10 to 15 ml of thick, yellow secretions with each session. The patient has a good cough effort and his breath sounds continue to reveal crackles in the right middle lobe. A repeat chest radiograph is ordered for the next morning, and his fever is controlled with acetaminophen. Based on this information, what would you recommend and why?

91. Mr. Gonsalves was admitted for pneumonia and dehydration. Explain how the complication of dehydration would influence your assessment 24 hours after starting postural drainage on the patient.

92. Mr. Gonsalves has developed bacteremia and has been transferred to the ICU. You determine Mr. Gonsalves will still benefit from postural drainage and percussion. During his initial treatment, you notice a dysrhythmia on the ECG monitor. Explain what you should do.

POSTTEST

1. Which of the following is *not* a goal of chest physical therapy according to the AARC Clinical Practice Guidelines?

   a. promote a more efficient breathing pattern
   b. improve distribution of ventilation
   c. restore a patient's PFT values to predicted range
   d. improve cardiopulmonary exercise tolerance

2. Your patient has been admitted for aspiration pneumonia in the right middle lobe. How would you position this patient for postural drainage?

   a. head down 15°, supine
   b. head down 15°, lying on the left side, rotated 1/4 turn backward
   c. head down 30°, lying on left side
   d. head down 20°, rotated 1/2 turn forward, lying on right side

3. Which of the following is considered an absolute contraindication to postural drainage?

   a. unstable head and neck injury
   b. empyema
   c. increased intracranial pressure
   d. lung contusion

4. *Haemophilus influenzae* pneumonia is characterized by sputum that is:

   a. rusty and thin.
   b. apple-green and thick.
   c. similar to red currant jelly.
   d. pink, thin, and blood-streaked.

5. Segments of the right upper lobe include:

   I.   apical.
   II. medial.
   III. posterior.
   IV. anterior.

      a. IV only
      b. I and III only
      c. I, III, and IV only
      d. all of the above

6. Which of the following slow ciliary activity?

   I.   excessive mucus production
   II. drying of the respiratory mucosa
   III. atropine
   IV. stimulation of the parasympathetic nervous system

      a. I and II only
      b. III and IV only
      c. I, II, and III only
      d. all of the above

7. High-frequency chest wall compression is best described as:

    a. a mechanical technique for augmenting secretion clearance using an oscillating vest.
    b. percussion of the chest using a hand-held motorized device.
    c. application of mechanical pressure to the epigastric region or thoracic cage.
    d. rapid vibration to the lateral costal margins on inspiration.

8. An elderly patient is seen in the clinic with a complaint of shortness of breath. The patient's history reveals a longstanding condition of pulmonary emphysema. On examination you observe the patient has short, shallow, gasping respirations at a rapid rate. He is using accessory muscles and appears anxious. Breathing exercises and coaching are:

    a. indicated to decrease the $PaCO_2$ levels.
    b. not indicated because the patient needs postural drainage.
    c. indicated because this type of coaching will help the patient control his breathing and decrease the work of breathing.
    d. not indicated because the problem is psychological and cannot be treated effectively in the clinic.

9. Which of the following is/are advantages of pursed lip breathing?

    I.   Tachypnea is reduced.
    II. The respiratory rate may decrease.
    III. Small airways remain open during exhalation.
    IV. The patient can gain control over his or her breathing.

        a. I and III only
        b. II and IV only
        c. I, II, and IV only
        d. all of the above

10. Techniques used to improve the strength and endurance of respiratory muscles include:

    I.   postural drainage.
    II. inspiratory resistive breathing.
    III. autogenic drainage.
    IV. PEP mask therapy.
    V. diaphragmatic breathing.

        a. II and V only
        b. I, III, and IV only
        c. I, II, and IV only
        d. IV and V only

11. With PEP therapy the patient is taught to actively, but not forcefully, exhale through a flow resistor to maintain a:

    a. positive pressure between 10 and 20 cm H_2O.
    b. resistive load of 30%.
    c. flowrate of 60 to 80 liters per minute.
    d. small but constant leak.

12. Mechanisms impairing the cough reflex include which of the following?

    I.   abdominal restriction
    II. narcotic analgesics
    III. anesthesia
    IV. neuromuscular dysfunction

        a. I and II only
        b. III and IV only
        c. II, III, and IV only
        d. all of the above

13. The phases of an effective cough include:

    I.   inspiration.
    II. irritation.
    III. expulsion.
    IV. compression.

        a. I, III, and IV only
        b. I and III only
        c. II and IV only
        d. all of the above

14. Necrotizing pneumonia is characterized by radiographic features demonstrating:

    a. Kerley lines.
    b. confluent shadows.
    c. cavities.
    d. air-bronchogram effect.

15. The most common disorder caused by RSV is:

    a. bronchiolitis.
    b. mycosis.
    c. asthmatic bronchitis.
    d. ARDS.

16. Indications for turning (continuous lateral rotational therapy) include:

    I.   immobility.
    II. presence of an artificial airway.
    III. presence of atelectasis.
    IV. poor oxygenation associated with position.

        a. I and IV only
        b. II, III, and IV only
        c. I, II, and III only
        d. all of the above

17. Benefits patients experience once they have been taught and use relaxation positioning include which of the following?

    I.   Proper positioning relaxes the abdominal muscles, allowing for better descent of the diaphragm.
    II. Upper arm positioning allows the patient more efficient use of the accessory muscles of inspiration.
    III. Resistive load is decreased by 30%.
    IV. Expiratory gas flow is effectively increased, decreasing trapped gas.

    a. I and III only
    b. I and II only
    c. II, III, and IV only
    d. all of the above

18. Inspiratory resistive breathing devices are designed primarily to improve the strength and endurance of the:

    a. accessory muscles of inspiration.
    b. accessory muscles of expiration.
    c. diaphragm.
    d. abdominal muscles.

19. Infection control practices employed during chest physical therapy would include which of the following?

    I.   implementing universal precautions
    II. observing all infection control guidelines posted for the patient
    III. disinfecting all equipment used between patients

    a. I only
    b. II only
    c. III only
    d. all of the above

20. According to the AARC Clinical Practice Guidelines for Postural Drainage Therapy, indications for postural drainage include:

    I.   difficulty clearing secretions with expectorated sputum greater than 25 to 30 ml/day.
    II. presence of foreign body in the airway.
    III. presence of atelectasis caused by, or suspected of being caused by, mucus plugging.
    IV. dyspnea experienced in the upright position.

    a. I and II only
    b. I and III only
    c. I, II, and III only
    d. all of the above

21. The PEP technique is best described as the patient:

    I. exhaling against a fixed-orifice flow resistor.
    II. inhaling against a fixed-orifice flow resistor.
    III. applying pressure on the diaphragm during inspiration.
    IV. creating a positive expiratory pressure by pursing his or her lips.

       a. II only
       b. III only
       c. I only
       d. IV only

22. Clinical situations indicating the need for the directed cough technique include:

    I. presence of atelectasis.
    II. spontaneous cough that fails to clear secretions.
    III. postoperative upper abdominal or thoracic surgery.
    IV. presence of reduced coronary artery perfusion.

       a. I and III only
       b. I, II, and III only
       c. II, III, and IV only
       d. all of the above

23. Contraindications for percussion and vibration include:

    I. recent skin grafts.
    II. subcutaneous emphysema.
    III. bronchospasm.
    IV. coagulopathy.

       a. I and IV only
       b. II and III only
       c. I, II, and III only
       d. all of the above

24. Parameters that should be monitored during postural drainage include:

    I. arterial oxygen saturation.
    II. breath sounds.
    III. heart rate and rhythm.
    IV. breathing rate and pattern.

       a. I and IV only
       b. III and IV only
       c. II, III, and IV only
       d. all of the above

25. Pneumococcal pneumonia is caused by:

    a. *Streptococcus pneumoniae.*
    b. *Pneumococcus pneumoniae.*
    c. *Klebsiella pneumoniae.*
    d. *Hemophilus pneumoniae.*

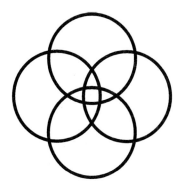

Volume Expansion

Resources

American Association for Respiratory Care: Clinical practice guideline: incentive spirometry, Resp Care 36:1402-1405, 1991.

American Association for Respiratory Care: Clinical practice guideline: intermittent positive pressure breathing, Resp Care 38:1189-1195, 1993.

American Association for Respiratory Care: Clinical practice guideline: use of positive airway pressure adjuncts to bronchial hygiene therapy, Resp Care 38:516-521, 1993.

Barnes TA: Core textbook of respiratory care practice, ed 2, St. Louis, 1994, Mosby.

Maas M, Buckwalter KC, and Hardy M: Nursing diagnoses and interventions for the elderly, Redwood City, CA, 1991, Addison-Wesley Nursing.

Scanlan CL, Spearman CB, and Sheldon RL, editors: Egan's fundamentals of respiratory care, ed 6, St. Louis, 1995, Mosby.

Topic 1: Pathophysiology of Atelectasis

1. Discuss the two pathogenic mechanisms associated with the development of atelectasis.

2. What are some of the risk factors or clinical conditions associated with the development of postoperative pulmonary complications like atelectasis and pneumonia?

3. What are the clinical signs associated with atelectasis?

4. What are the physiologic manifestations of atelectasis?

5. Discuss the age-related physiologic changes that contribute to the development of postoperative atelectasis and/or pneumonia.

6. State the spirometric values that indicate risk and high risk for postoperative pulmonary complications.

Spirometric Indicators of Risk and High Risk for Postoperative Pulmonary Complications*

Measurement	At Risk	At High Risk
FVC		
FEV_1		
FEV1		
FEV_1/FVC		
$FEF_{25\%-75\%}$		
MVV		

*FVC = forced vital capacity; FEV_1 = forced expiratory volume in 1 second; $FEF_{25\%-75\%}$ = forced expiratory flow, midexpiratory phase; MVV = maximal voluntary ventilation.

Table 4-1 From Barnes TA: Core textbook of respiratory care practice, ed 2, St. Louis, 1994, Mosby.

True/False

7. **T F** Advanced age, smoking history, general debilitation, and malnutrition are considered risk factors for developing postoperative pulmonary complications.

8. **T F** An abnormal sigh mechanism can result in the development of atelectasis.

9. **T F** Increased radiopacity, diminished lung volume, and hilar displacement are all chest radiograph findings characteristic of atelectasis.

10. **T F** Increases in lung compliance, functional residual capacity, and work of breathing are considered to be physiologic manifestations of atelectasis.

11. **T F** Chest physical examination findings consistent with the diagnosis of atelectasis include decreased chest expansion, dull percussion note, tactile fremitus, and diminished breath sounds.

12. **T F** With significant atelectasis, the mediastinum may be shifted away from the atelectatic lung.

▬ Topic 2: Incentive Spirometry ▬▬▬▬▬▬▬▬▬▬▬

13. Describe the physiologic basis for having patients perform repeated sustained maximal inspiration maneuvers.

14. Describe the indications for incentive spirometry.

15. What are the contraindications to incentive spirometry?

16. List the hazards and complications of incentive spirometry.

17. Discuss the advantages of performing preoperative incentive spirometry teaching and assessment.

18. Discuss incentive spirometry patient teaching including a description of the technique and goal setting.

19. Discuss patient monitoring and follow-up performed with incentive spirometry therapy.

20. Describe the incentive spirometry outcome assessment for atelectasis and improved muscle performance.

21. How are the two incentive spirometry devices pictured below different?

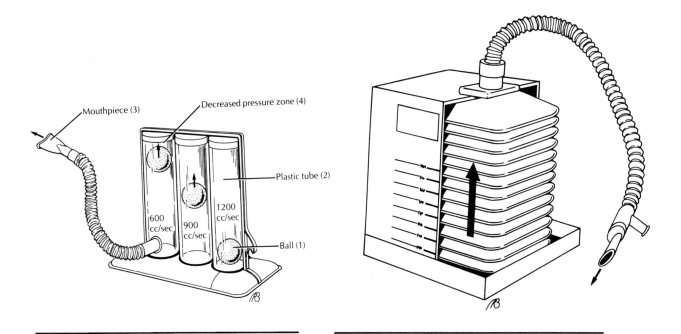

Figure 4-1a   From Eubanks DH and Bone RC: Comprehensive respiratory care: a learning system, ed 2, St. Louis, 1990, Mosby.

Figure 4-1b   From Eubanks DH and Bone RC: Comprehensive respiratory care: a learning system, ed 2, St. Louis, 1990, Mosby.

22. Calculate the estimated inspiratory volume for a patient using a flow-oriented incentive spirometer at a flow of 1200 cc/sec with an inspiratory hold of 3 seconds.

True/False

23. **T F**   When incentive spirometry is performed too rapidly, the most common patient complaint is dizziness.

24. **T F**   When using flow-oriented incentive spirometry devices, flow is equated with volume by this formula: flow **x** inspiratory time = volume.

25. **T F**   Flow-oriented devices are superior to volume-oriented incentive devices.

26. **T F**   During the preliminary planning for an incentive spirometry trial, the therapeutic outcomes should be set.

27. **T F**   Universal precautions must be followed as outlined by the CDC with all incentive spirometry treatments.

▰ Topic 3: Intermittent Positive Pressure Breathing ▰▰▰▰▰▰

28. Discuss the physiologic basis for IPPB therapy.

29. Discuss the indications for IPPB therapy.

30. According to the AARC Clinical Practice Guideline for IPPB therapy, what are the contraindications for IPPB therapy?

31. According to the AARC Clinical Practice Guideline for IPPB therapy, what are the complications and hazards of IPPB therapy?

32. Discuss the baseline assessment of patients prior to initiating IPPB therapy.

33. What patient outcomes indicate successful IPPB therapy?

34. What infection control precautions should be followed when administering IPPB therapy?

35. What patient parameters would you monitor while performing IPPB therapy?

36. Describe the machine parameters you would monitor while performing IPPB therapy.

37. When performing volume-oriented IPPB, how is the goal volume determined?

True/False

38. **T F**   The optimal breathing pattern for IPPB therapy is slow, deep breaths that are sustained or held at end-inspiration.

39. **T F**   Patients with fatigue or muscle weakness resulting in impending respiratory failure are not candidates for IPPB trials.

40. **T F**   IPPB therapy is considered beneficial when the IPPB tidal volume is greater than the spontaneous tidal volume by at least 25%.

41. **T F**   IPPB therapy has been shown to augment tidal volume and increase minute ventilation, thereby lowering the arterial PCO_2 in patients with acute hypercapnic respiratory failure.

42. **T F**   Incorrectly applied IPPB can be a less effective method of aerosol administration when compared to simpler methods, even in patients with suboptimal breathing patterns.

43. **T F**   Active hemoptysis is considered a contraindication for IPPB therapy because the positive pressure may worsen the situation.

44. **T F**   Coaching patients to keep their respiratory rate between 6 and 8 breaths/minute during IPPB therapy can decrease the risk of hypocapnia and respiratory alkalosis.

45. **T F**   IPPB therapy enhances venous return and cardiac output.

46. **T F**   IPPB can cause or worsen air trapping, which can increase the risk of pulmonary barotrauma.

47. **T F**   The best way to avoid air trapping with IPPB is to use high flowrates and encourage high respiratory rates.

48. **T F**   Patients should be placed in as close to an upright position as possible for IPPB treatments.

49. **T F**   Initial settings for IPPB therapy include sensitivity of -1 to -2 cm H_2O and system pressure between 10 to 15 cm H_2O.

50. **T F**   When treating atelectasis, volume-oriented outcomes should be used, such as achieving a tidal volume of 10 to 15 ml/kg or at least 30% of the patient's predicted inspiratory capacity.

51. **T F**   When system pressure drops after inspiration begins or fails to rise until the end of the patient breath during IPPB, the problem is incorrect setting of the sensitivity.

52. **T F**   Hazards of IPPB therapy include gastric distention, hypoventilation, and mismatch of ventilation and perfusion.

Topic 4: Positive Airway Pressure Breathing

53. What is positive airway pressure therapy (PAP)?

54. Describe expiratory positive airway pressure (EPAP), positive expiratory pressure (PEP), and continuous positive airway pressure (CPAP).

55. What are the indications for PAP therapy?

56. What are the contraindications for PAP therapy?

57. List the hazards and complications associated with PAP therapy.

58. Discuss the assessment of need for PAP therapy.

59. According to the AARC Clinical Practice Guidelines for PAP as adjunct to bronchial hygiene therapy, describe the assessment of outcome.

60. What basic equipment is needed for PEP, CPAP, and EPAP therapy?

61. Discuss the monitoring of patients requiring PAP therapy.

True/False

62. **T F** Positive airway pressure adjuncts are used to mobilize secretions and treat atelectasis.

63. **T F** During CPAP therapy, the patient breathes from a pressurized circuit that maintains pressures between 20 and 50 cm H_2O during inspiration and expiration.

64. **T F** PEP therapy generates pressures during expiration of 10 to 20 cm H_2O using fixed-orifice resistors.

65. **T F** PEP therapy and EPAP therapy produce the same mechanical and physiologic effects.

66. **T F** EPAP therapy incorporates the use of a threshold resistor to create pressures on exhalation of 10 to 20 cm H_2O.

▬ Topic 5: Follow-up to Mrs. Howell ▬▬▬▬▬▬▬▬▬▬

Refer to the therapist-driven protocol on page 208 to answer the following.

67. Because Mrs. Howell's actual inspiratory capacity was less than 80% of predicted, she was started on supervised incentive spirometry every four hours with an automatic reevaluation at 24 hours. After 24 hours, her inspiratory capacity was approximately 1.30 liters compared to her predicted value of 1.55 liters. She was coughing well with assistance in splinting. What would you recommend?

68. On the first day of incentive spirometry therapy, Mrs. Howell was averaging inspired volumes of 1.0 liter. After 24 hours of therapy, she was averaging inspiratory volumes of 1.1 liters. She is coughing well with assistance and a great deal of coaching. She is afebrile and her breath sounds are clear but diminished at the bases because of the abdominal binder. What would you recommend?

69. Twenty-four hours after the incentive spirometry was initiated, Mrs. Howell shows no improvement in her inspiratory volumes, her breath sounds indicate retained secretions, and her cough is weak and ineffective in clearing the secretions. She now has a fever of 101° F. What would you recommend?

70. Four days postop, Mrs. Howell's volumes with the incentive spirometer meet her preoperative inspiratory capacity volume. She works well with the device between visits from the respiratory care practitioner, and she has a strong cough and is afebrile. What would you recommend?

1. Assessment outcomes designed to evaluate the resolution of or reduction in signs of atelectasis following the initiation of incentive spirometry include:

   I.   improvement in previously absent or diminished breath sounds.
   II. return of FRC or VC to preoperative values.
   III. return to normal chest radiograph.
   IV. resolution of fever and normalization of vital signs.

      a. I, II, and IV only
      b. I and III only
      c. I, III, and IV only
      d. all of the above

2. As you treat a patient with IPPB, he complains of dizziness and a tingling sensation in his fingertips. Which of the following is the most likely cause?

      a. fatigue
      b. alveolar hyperventilation
      c. decreased cardiac output
      d. increased intracranial pressure

3. Which of the following conditions are considered to be relative contraindication(s) to positive airway pressure therapies such as CPAP, PEP, and EPAP?

   I.   esophageal surgery
   II. hemoptysis
   III. increased intracranial pressure
   IV. atelectasis

      a. I, II, and IV only
      b. I, II, and III only
      c. I, III, and IV only
      d. all of the above

4. Goals of positive airway pressure therapy include:

   I.   reduction of air trapping in asthma and COPD.
   II. mobilization of retained secretions.
   III. prevention or reversal of atelectasis.
   IV. improvement of the pacing of the diaphragm.

      a. I and II only
      b. III and IV only
      c. I, II, and III only
      d. all of the above

5. Pulmonary Function Test results indicating increased risk of postoperative pulmonary complications include:

    I.   FVC less than 50% of predicted.
    II. FEV_1 less than 50% of predicted.
    III. $FEF_{25\%-75\%}$; less than 50% of predicted.
    IV. FEV_1/FVC less than 50%.

    a. IV only
    b. I and III only
    c. I, III, and IV only
    d. all of the above

6. Physiologic signs associated with atelectasis include:

    I.   excessive mucus production.
    II. reduced lung compliance.
    III. increased shunting.
    IV. increased FRC.

    a. I and II only
    b. III and IV only
    c. II and III only
    d. all of the above

7. The best way to avoid air trapping during IPPB is to allow sufficient time for exhalation by:

    a. letting the patient choose a rate that is comfortable.
    b. using low rates (6 to 8/min.) and long expiratory times.
    c. using low rates (6 to 8/min.) and short expiratory times.
    d. using rapid rates (14 to 16/min.) and long expiratory times.

8. The most common problem associated with administering positive airway pressure therapies is:

    a. leaks in the system.
    b. a lack of understanding by the patient.
    c. the malfunctioning of equipment.
    d. the necessity of cleaning the equipment.

9. An assessment of need for incentive spirometry should be completed on patients with:

    I.   neuromuscular disease involving respiratory musculature.
    II. poor pain control and immobility.
    III. surgical procedures involving the thorax.
    IV. surgical procedures involving the upper abdomen.

    a. I and III only
    b. II and IV only
    c. I, II, and IV only
    d. all of the above

10. Clinical situations contraindicating incentive spirometry include:

    I.   one or more chest tubes in place.
    II. IC less than 1/3 of predicted.
    III. VC less than 10 ml/kg.
    IV. dysfunctional diaphragm.

        a. II and III only
        b. I, III, and IV only
        c. I, II, and IV only
        d. I and IV only

11. With PEP therapy, the patient is taught to actively, but not forcefully, exhale through a flow resistor to maintain a:

        a. positive pressure between 0 and 80 cm H_2O.
        b. resistive load of 30%.
        c. 60 to 80 liters per minute expiratory flowrate.
        d. positive pressure between 10 and 20 cm H_2O.

12. Active tuberculosis should be considered a possible contraindication for IPPB therapy because:

    I.   IPPB may spread the localized infection.
    II. these patients are always hemodynamically unstable.
    III. the cavities seen in advanced stages of TB could rupture.
    IV. it is associated with increased airway resistance.

        a. I and II only
        b. I and III only
        c. II, III, and IV only
        d. all of the above

13. Before administering volume expansion therapy of any kind, patient teaching should include an explanation of which of the following?

    I.   why the therapy has been ordered
    II. what the therapy does
    III. how the therapy will feel
    IV. what the expected results are

        a. I, III, and IV only
        b. I and III only
        c. II and IV only
        d. all of the above

14. In the diagram below, the solid lines are alveolar pressures and the dotted lines are pleural pressures. Side A represents spontaneous breathing. What does side B represent?

    a. EPAP
    b. CPAP
    c. IPPB
    d. PEP

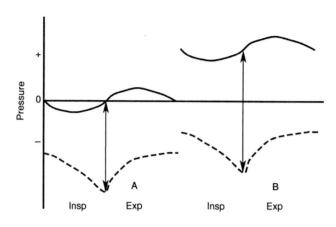

Figure 4-2 From Scanlan CL, Spearman CB, and Sheldon RL, editors: Egan's fundamentals of respiratory care, ed 6, St. Louis, 1995, Mosby.

15. All of the following are considered clinical signs of atelectasis *except*:

    a. hyperresonant percussion note.
    b. decreased chest excursion.
    c. fever with pneumonitis.
    d. diminished breath sounds.

16. Benefits of CPAP therapy as a treatment for cardiogenic pulmonary edema include:

    I.   increased venous return.
    II. reduced cardiac filling pressures.
    III. improved lung compliance.
    IV. decreased work of breathing.

        a. I and IV only
        b. II, III, and IV only
        c. I, II, and III only
        d. all of the above

17. Current approaches to positive airway pressure therapy include:

    I.   expiratory positive airway pressure (EPAP).
    II. continuous positive airway pressure (CPAP).
    III. zero end-expiratory pressure (ZEEP).
    IV. positive expiratory pressure (PEP).

        a. I, II, and IV only
        b. I and II only
        c. II, III, and IV only
        d. all of the above

18. The AARC Clinical Practice Guideline for intermittent positive pressure breathing suggests an assessment outcome for IPPB to be an increase in tidal volume of at least _____ % during therapy compared to the pretreatment spontaneous tidal volume.

    a. 10
    b. 15
    c. 25
    d. 35

19. Infection control practices implemented by respiratory care practitioners with IPPB therapy would include which of the following?

    I. following all universal precautions
    II. observing all infection control guidelines posted for the patient
    III. disinfecting all reusable equipment between patients
    IV. rinsing nebulizers with tap water between treatments

        a. I and II only
        b. II and IV only
        c. I, II, and III only
        d. all of the above

20. When selecting the best method for achieving a given clinical goal, the volume expansion therapy chosen should be:

    I. safe.
    II. simple to use.
    III. effective.
    IV. disposable.

        a. I, II, and III only
        b. I and III only
        c. I, II, and IV only
        d. all of the above

21. Relative contraindications to IPPB therapy include all of the following *except*:

    a. active hemoptysis.
    b. hypocarbia.
    c. radiographic evidence of bleb.
    d. active untreated tuberculosis.

22. Your patient has just completed her first incentive spirometry session, and she complains of dizziness and slight tingling in her fingers. Your initial response would be to:

    a. call her physician immediately to discontinue the therapy.
    b. check her fingers and forehead for cyanosis.
    c. encourage her to relax and breathe quietly for a few minutes.
    d. call her physician to change her to CPAP therapy.

23. Monitoring of patients during positive airway pressure therapy should include the evaluation of:

    I.   respiratory rate and pattern.
    II. sputum color, amount, consistency, and odor.
    III. pulse rate and rhythm.
    IV. breath sounds.

    a. I and IV only
    b. II and III only
    c. I, II, and III only
    d. all of the above

24. Hazards/complications of positive airway pressure adjuncts used to mobilize secretions and treat atelectasis include:

    I.   claustrophobia.
    II. pulmonary barotrauma.
    III. increased intracranial pressure.
    IV. cardiovascular compromise.

    a. I and IV only
    b. III and IV only
    c. II, III, and IV only
    d. all of the above

25. You are administering an IPPB treatment with 0.5 cc of Proventil (albuterol) QID to a 60-year-old, 70-kilogram female patient who is recovering from thoracic surgery. Her current spontaneous vital capacity is 0.60 L. During the treatment she consistently achieves volumes of 0.85 L, with a cycling pressure of 16 cm H_2O. Based on this information, what would you do?

    a. Increase the cycling pressure and evaluate the new tidal volume.
    b. Discontinue the IPPB and initiate incentive spirometry QID.
    c. Discontinue the IPPB and change to EPAP therapy.
    d. Continue the therapy at 15 cm H_2O and assess next session.

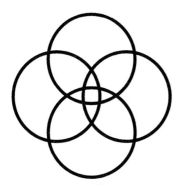

Physical Assessment

Resources

Barnes TA: Core textbook of respiratory care practice, ed 2, St. Louis, 1994, Mosby.

Scanlan CL, Spearman CB, and Sheldon RL, editors: Egan's fundamentals of respiratory care, ed 6, St. Louis, 1995, Mosby.

Wilkins RL, Krider SJ, and Sheldon RL, editors: Clinical assessment in respiratory care, ed 3, St. Louis, 1995, Mosby.

Topic 1: Initial Patient Assessment and History

1. What is the purpose of the patient interview portion of a patient assessment?

2. In order to conduct a successful interview, skill and professional etiquette come into play. Describe guidelines the RCP should keep in mind while conducting patient interviews.

3. What is a chief complaint?

4. What information would you attempt to gather when questioning patients regarding their present illnesses?

5. Why is it important to notice the patient's overall appearance and to determine an initial impression of your patient when conducting a physical examination interview?

6. How is sensorium evaluated?

7. What information is gained by observing a patient's facial expression?

8. Prepare an outline of the general items you would include when developing a patient history.

9. Describe the four parts of the Weed system of patient evaluation.

True/False

10. **T F**   A chief complaint should not be recorded until verified by laboratory data.

11. **T F**   Family history usually includes the age and health, or age and cause of death, of each immediate family member.

12. **T F**   When acquiring patients' psychosocial histories, it may be important to question them on their cultural or religious beliefs relevant to perceptions of health, illness, and treatment.

13. **T F**   Childhood illnesses such as scarlet fever, rubella, and poliomyelitis have little relevance to the medical history of adult patients since many years have passed and treatment has improved.

14. **T F**   When interviewing patients, it is important to show your respect for their personal beliefs, attitudes, and rights.

▮ Topic 2: Vital Signs ▮

15. State the normal body temperature for adults.

16. What effect does fever have on oxygen consumption and carbon dioxide production?

17. Explain why a patient with hypothermia might exhibit decreases in respiratory rate and heart rate.

18. What is an adult's normal pulse rate?

19. What is pulsus paradoxus and when is it seen?

20. State the normal resting respiratory rate for adults.

21. Give three examples of diseases, conditions, or patient situations that can result in bradypnea.

22. State the normal adult blood pressure.

23. Define hypotension and give three causes.

24. Define hypertension and state the most common cause.

25. List three mistakes in blood pressure measurement technique that can result in falsely high blood pressure readings.

True/False

26. **T F**   A falsely high blood pressure reading can occur when the cuff is too wide for the patient's arm.

27. **T F**   A normal pulse pressure is 40 to 80 mm Hg.

28. **T F**   Proper placement of a blood pressure cuff is approximately one inch above the antecubital fossa.

29. **T F**   The pulse should be evaluated for rate, rhythm, amplitude, and other palpable vibrations.

30. **T F**   Oral temperatures are valid in patients breathing heated or cool aerosol via face mask.

31. **T F**   Prolonged hypotension can result in impaired oxygen delivery and tissue hypoxia.

32. **T F**   Pulsus alternans may be seen in left heart failure and is denoted by a beat-to-beat variability in pulse amplitude.

33. **T F**   Pulsus paradoxus can be exhibited in acute asthma, chronic obstructive pulmonary disease, and cardiac tamponade.

34. **T F**   A bounding pulse is characteristic of cardiac disease, shock, and hypotension.

35. **T F**   Tachycardia may be seen in patients with fever, hypoxia, anxiety, and shock.

▬ Topic 3: Chest Physical Assessment ▬▬▬▬▬▬▬

36. Briefly describe the following chest abnormalities: barrel chest, funnel chest, pigeon chest, scoliosis, and kyphosis.

37. When performing the inspection phase of a physical assessment, give five examples of things you are observing.

38. What is abdominal paradox, and when is it seen?

39. What is respiratory alternans, and when is it seen?

40. What is palpation, and what is its purpose?

41. What is percussion?

42. Give two examples each of (1) diseases or conditions that produce dull percussion sounds and (2) diseases or conditions that produce hyperresonant percussion sounds.

43. Describe common errors made while performing auscultation of the chest.

44. Diagram vesicular, bronchovesicular, and bronchial breath sounds, and state where these sounds are normally heard.

45. Differentiate between wheezes and crackles.

46. Describe a pleural friction rub.

47. What is whispering pectoriloquy, and what advantage does it offer over simple auscultation of the chest?

48. Describe stridor and give three causes.

49. How is capillary refill assessed?

50. What is clubbing of the digits?

True/False

51. **T F** Men and women breathe the same way; both use a combination of intercostal muscles and the diaphragm, producing mostly chest movement with inspiration.

52. **T F** Cyanosis is the first sign of hypoxia.

53. **T F** Palpation of the chest over an area of pneumonia or consolidation reveals decreased fremitus.

54. **T F** Normal resonance is the term used to describe the sound heard over the normal air-filled lung during percussion.

55. **T F** Diaphragmatic excursion is assessed by palpation.

56. **T F** Normal diaphragmatic excursion during deep breathing is approximately 5 to 7 cm.

57. **T F** It is best to percuss the entire left chest top to bottom before percussing the right side.

58. **T F** A crackling sound and sensation is palpated over subcutaneous emphysema.

59. **T F** Patients who are obese or overly muscular often demonstrate a reduced tactile fremitus during palpation.

60. **T F** Peripheral cyanosis is most often related to poor circulation.

Matching

Match the definition on the right to the type of breathing pattern on the left.

61. _____ Biot's   **A.** absence of breathing

62. _____ Kussmaul's   **B.** prolonged exhalation

63. _____ Cheyne-Stokes   **C.** irregular breathing with periods of apnea

64. _____ apneustic   **D.** rapid, deep breathing

65. _____ apnea   **E.** breaths that increase in volume, then decrease in volume, with periods of apnea

                          F. prolonged inhalation

Fill in the Blank

66. Complete the following table by providing the common palpation, percussion, and auscultation findings.

Abnormality	Initial Impression	Inspection	Palpation	Percussion	Auscultation	Possible Causes
Acute airway obstruction	Appears acutely ill	Use of accessory muscles				Asthma, bronchitis
Chronic airway obstruction	Appears chronically ill	Increased anteroposterior diameter, use of accessory muscles				Chronic bronchitis, emphysema
Consolidation	May appear acutely ill	Inspiratory lag				Pneumonia, tumor
Pneumothorax	May appear acutely ill	Unilateral expansion				Rib fracture, open wound
Pleural effusion	May appear acutely ill	Unilateral expansion				Congestive heart failure
Local bronchial obstruction	Appears acutely ill	Unilateral expansion				Mucous plug
Diffuse interstitial fibrosis	Often normal	Rapid shallow breathing				Chronic exposure to inorganic dust
Acute upper airway obstruction	Appears acutely ill	Labored breathing				Epiglottitis, croup, foreign body aspiration

From Wilkins RL, Krider SJ, and Sheldon RL, editors: Clinical assessment in respiratory care, ed 3, St. Louis, 1995, Mosby.

▰ Topic 4: Chest Trauma ▰▰▰▰▰▰▰▰▰▰

67. Describe the signs and symptoms of a pneumothorax.

68. What is a tension pneumothorax?

69. What is a pneumomediastinum, and when does it develop?

70. What is a pleural effusion?

71. Describe the signs and symptoms associated with a pleural effusion.

72. Describe paradoxical (flail) chest wall movement.

73. What is subcutaneous emphysema, when does it occur, and how is it identified?

True/False

74. **T F** Blood in the pleural space is called a *hemothorax.*

75. **T F** Paradoxical chest wall movement is seen with all rib fractures.

76. **T F** The most common symptoms associated with a pleural effusion are dyspnea, pleuritic chest pain, and a dry, nonproductive cough.

77. **T F** The mediastinum moves away from the affected side when a tension pneumothorax is present.

78. **T F** Asymmetric chest movement is characteristic of unilateral pulmonary disease processes.

Topic 5: Chest Drainage

79. Describe the purpose of closed chest drainage.

80. When is chest drainage indicated?

81. Identify the device pictured below, and describe its use.

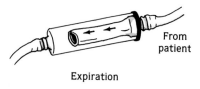

Expiration

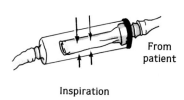

Inspiration

Figure 5-1 From Wilkins RL, Krider SJ, and Sheldon RL, editors: Clinical assessment in respiratory care, ed 3, St. Louis, 1995, Mosby.

B

82. What is the purpose of the water seal chamber of a chest drainage system?

83. Differentiate between continuous bubbling, intermittent bubbling, and absent bubbling in the water seal chamber.

84. What is the purpose of the collection chamber of closed-chest drainage systems?

85. What is the purpose of the suction control chamber of closed-chest drainage systems?

86. Identify the components of the three-bottle chest drainage system pictured below.

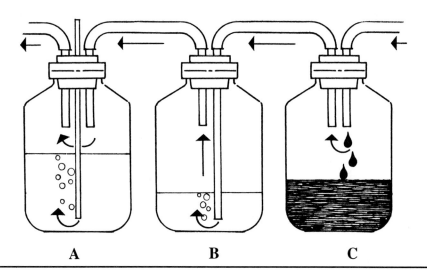

A   B   C

Figure 5-2 Courtesy of Atrium Medical Corporation, Hudson, New Hampshire.

True/False

87. **T F**   An improperly functioning chest drainage system can add air or fluid to the pleural space.

88. **T F**   Most commonly, the suction control chamber is filled to 20 cm H_2O.

89. **T F**   Free-flowing, bright-red, warm blood draining at a rate of 500 to 1000 ml/hr is common following chest tube insertion and is of no real concern.

90. **T F**   It is common to leave chest tubes in place, until there is no air leak with a cough for 24 to 48 hours.

91. **T F**   Following lung surgery, it is common to see a brief, sudden increase in dark, bloody drainage through the chest tube when the patient is turned.

Topic 6: Assessment of the Trauma Patient

92. When assessing a trauma patient for the first time, what is assessed first, and how is this accomplished?

93. Describe how you would determine if a patient's airway is partially or totally occluded.

94. List four causes of airway obstruction.

95. How is an obstructed airway opened in a trauma patient?

96. Describe the assessment of breathing in the trauma patient.

97. Describe the assessment of circulation in the trauma patient.

98. Explain why trauma patients are at risk for decreased oxygen delivery to tissues such as the brain and kidneys.

■ Topic 7: Follow-up to Mr. Donovan ▨▨▨▨▨▨▨▨▨▨▨▨▨▨▨▨▨▨▨▨

Refer to the therapist-driven protocol on page 209 to complete the following.

99. Mr. Donovan is receiving oxygen from a non-rebreather mask when you begin your assessment. As you assess his airway, you notice he stops breathing. What should you do?

100. During your initial assessment of Mr. Donovan, you determine his airway is obstructed. Describe your actions.

101. You deliver oxygen to Mr. Donovan with a non-rebreather mask, and his pulse oximetry reads 98% saturation after 30 minutes. His pulse and respiratory rate are increased, he is confused, and his capillary refill is at least 5 seconds. You check his chart and find he has had no urine output. What would you suggest?

POSTTEST

1. Which of the following is consistent with fever?

   a. decreased respiratory rate
   b. acrocyanosis
   c. decreased heart rate
   d. increased oxygen consumption

2. Adult hypotension is defined as a blood pressure less than:

   a. 140/90.
   b. 90/60.
   c. 100/75.
   d. 120/80.

3. When called to evaluate a multiple trauma patient in the emergency department, the respiratory care practitioner should first assess the:

   a. airway to determine patency.
   b. heart rate and blood pressure to determine adequacy of circulation.
   c. character of respirations.
   d. level of consciousness.

4. Paradoxical chest wall movement is best described as:

   a. the inward movement of the chest on inspiration and the outward movement on expiration.
   b. the outward movement of the chest on inspiration and the inward movement on expiration.
   c. decreased movement on one side of the chest with normal movement on the opposite side.
   d. normal movement of the chest for a period of time followed by a period of abnormal movement.

5. Which of the following affect a person's ability to breathe spontaneously?

   I.   intact thoracic cage
   II. patent airway
   III. normal negative intrapleural pressure
   IV. intact nervous system control of ventilation

       a. IV only
       b. I and III only
       c. I, III, and IV only
       d. all of the above

6. Possible causes of abdominal paradox include:

   I.   respiratory muscle fatigue.
   II. splinting after abdominal surgery.
   III. diaphragmatic paralysis.
   IV. chronic obstructive pulmonary disease.

       a. I and II only
       b. III and IV only
       c. I, II, and III only
       d. all of the above

7. When auscultating a patient's chest, you determine that the spoken voice increases in intensity and its character takes on a nasal quality. This is referred to as:

    a. bronchophony.
    b. pectoriloquy.
    c. egophony.
    d. polyphony.

8. Breath sounds that are high-pitched with an expiratory component equal to or slightly longer than inspiration are best referred to as:

    a. bronchovesicular.
    b. bronchial.
    c. sonorous.
    d. stridorous.

9. Clinical signs of a decreased cardiac output include:

    I.   very warm and dry skin.
    II. decreased urine output (less than 0.5 ml/kg/hr).
    III. dizziness and syncope with position changes.
    IV. decreased mentation and altered level of consciousness.

        a. I, II, and III only
        b. II, III, and IV only
        c. I, II, and IV only
        d. all of the above

10. A patient's airway may be occluded by:

    I.   bilateral vocal cord paralysis.
    II. spasms of the larynx and bronchi.
    III. excessive secretions.
    IV. loss of tonicity of the submandibular muscles.

        a. II and IV only
        b. I, III, and IV only
        c. I, II, and IV only
        d. all of the above

11. Deep and fast breathing associated with metabolic acidosis is known as:

    a. Kussmaul's.
    b. Cheyne-Stokes.
    c. Biot's.
    d. asthmatic.

12. Continuous bubbling in the water seal chamber of a chest drainage system may indicate:

    I.   a large active pneumothorax.
    II. a leak in the system.
    III. variations in the suction control chamber.
    IV. a malfunction of the Heimlich valve.

        a. I and II only
        b. III and IV only
        c. II, III, and IV only
        d. all of the above

13. Palpation is a technique performed to:

    I.   assess the skin and subcutaneous tissue.
    II. evaluate vocal fremitus.
    III. estimate thoracic expansion.
    IV. assess central nervous system stimulation.

        a. I and II only
        b. I, II, and III only
        c. III and IV only
        d. I, II, and IV only

14. Tactile fremitus will be increased in all of the following *except*:

        a. atelectasis.
        b. pulmonary fibrosis.
        c. pleural effusion.
        d. pneumonia.

15. Lethargic patients are best described as:

        a. sleepy and easily aroused, answering appropriately when aroused and questioned.
        b. confused and easily agitated, exhibiting hallucinations.
        c. unresponsive to stimuli and not exhibiting voluntary movement.
        d. having slow mental responses and a dulled perception.

16. Clubbing of the digits is seen in patients with:

    I.   cystic fibrosis.
    II. bronchogenic carcinoma.
    III. bronchiectasis.
    IV. chest trauma.

        a. I and II only
        b. II and III only
        c. I, II, and III only
        d. all of the above

17. Physical signs of diffuse interstitial fibrosis include:

    I.   late-inspiratory crackles on auscultation.
    II. normal or increased fremitus on palpation.
    III. increased anteroposterior diameter on inspection.
    IV. increased resonance with percussion.

       a. I and III only
       b. I and II only
       c. II, III, and IV only
       d. all of the above

18. The purpose of the water seal chamber of a chest drainage system is to:

    a. hasten the removal of air and fluid from the intrapleural space.
    b. serve as a one-way valve, permitting air to leave the pleural space while preventing its reentry.
    c. store accumulated blood and fluid from the pleural space without increasing the patient's work of breathing.
    d. provide an area for the accurate measurement of evacuated pleural fluid.

19. Effective patient interviewing techniques include which of the following?

    I.   Make immediate eye contact with the patient.
    II. Stand during the interview to show you are in charge.
    III. Use questions and statements that demonstrate sincerity.
    IV. When meeting a patient, address the patient by title.

       a. I and II only
       b. I and III only
       c. I, III, and IV only
       d. all of the above

20. Information regarding the adequacy of circulation can be gathered by assessing:

    I.   pulse quality, rate, and location.
    II. capillary refill.
    III. skin color and temperature.
    IV. level of consciousness.

       a. I and II only
       b. I and III only
       c. I, II, and IV only
       d. all of the above

21. Being able to conduct a good patient interview is important because:

    I.   the interview sets the climate for all further interaction between you and the patient.
    II. the interview is the most common method used to obtain a patient's medical history.
    III. the interview provides information on which to base and assess treatment.
    IV. patients dislike completing forms.

       a. I and III only
       b. I, II, and III only
       c. II, III, and IV only
       d. all of the above

22. When gathering information regarding a patient's present illness, it is important to include:

    I.   aggravating and/or alleviating factors.
    II. associated manifestations.
    III. frequency and duration of the illness.
    IV. time of onset.

        a. I and IV only
        b. I, II, and III only
        c. II, III, and IV only
        d. all of the above

23. Physical assessment consistent with acute upper airway obstruction reveals:

    I.   inspection—labored breathing.
    II. auscultation—late inspiratory crackles.
    III. auscultation—inspiratory/expiratory stridor.
    IV. percussion—often normal.

        a. I and II only
        b. II and IV only
        c. I, III, and IV only
        d. III and IV only

24. Physical findings associated with a pneumothorax include:

    I.   hyperresonance with percussion.
    II. decreased fremitus.
    III. decreased breath sounds.
    IV. increased respiratory rate.

        a. I and III only
        b. II and IV only
        c. II, III, and IV only
        d. all of the above

25. Percussion over an area of consolidation reveals:

    a. a dull note.
    b. increased resonance.
    c. slight decrease in resonance.
    d. tympanic sound.

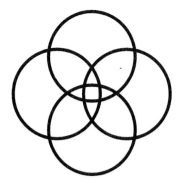

Pediatrics

Resources

American Association for Respiratory Care: Clinical practice guideline: bland aerosol administration, Resp Care 38:1196-1200, 1993.

American Association for Respiratory Care: Clinical practice guideline: selection of an aerosol delivery device for neonatal and pediatric patients, Resp Care 40:1325-1335, 1995.

Haley K, editor: Emergency nursing pediatric course (provider) manual, Chicago, 1993, Emergency Nurses Association.

Koff PB: Neonatal and pediatric respiratory care, ed 2, St. Louis, 1993, Mosby.

Turner J: Handbook of adult and pediatric respiratory home care, St. Louis, 1994, Mosby.

Wilkins RL, Krider SJ, and Sheldon RL, editors: Clinical assessment in respiratory care, ed 3, St. Louis, 1995, Mosby.

Wong DL: Whaley and Wong's nursing care of infants and children, ed 5, St. Louis, 1995, Mosby.

Topic 1: Croup and Epiglottitis

1. Briefly describe the three types of croup syndromes.

2. With what age range is classic croup most commonly associated?

3. Describe the clinical presentation of croup.

4. Describe the treatment of croup.

5. What is epiglottitis?

6. What causes epiglottitis?

7. Describe the classic clinical presentation of epiglottitis.

8. Describe the treatment of epiglottitis.

9. What is stridor?

10. Describe the relationship between the development of airway obstruction and the flow of gas through the airway. Include a description of how airway obstruction affects work of breathing.

True/False

11. **T F**   Epiglottitis is caused exclusively by respiratory syncytial virus.

12. **T F**   Croup is a common cause of upper airway obstruction in children that requires intubation in approximately 50% of the cases.

13. **T F**   Unlike classic croup, spasmodic croup has no seasonal predilection.

14. **T F**   Classic croup tends to recur in children susceptible to viral infections.

15. **T F**   The diagnosis of croup is usually based on the history provided, the physical findings, and, in some cases, radiograph findings.

16. **T F**   When children experience mild upper airway obstruction, they increase transthoracic pressure to achieve adequate air flow in and out of the lungs.

17. **T F**   Subglottic narrowing is present in laryngotracheobronchitis and supraglottic narrowing is present in epiglottitis.

18. **T F**   A child who presents with drooling and soft, low-pitched inspiratory stridor is best treated with racemic epinephrine.

19. **T F**   Lateral neck radiographs of a child with epiglottitis reveals ballooning of the hypopharynx, obliteration of the vallecula, edematous aryepiglottic folds, and an enlarged epiglottis.

20. **T F**   Lateral neck radiographs of a child with croup reveals subglottic narrowing, often called the steeple sign.

▬ Topic 2: Physiologic/Anatomical Pediatric Variations and ▬ the Care of the Pediatric Patient

21. Discuss the similarities and differences between children and adults with regard to mucus glands, alveoli, and the thoracic cage.

22. Explain why the pediatric airway is more susceptible to obstruction compared to the adult airway.

23. What are the normal respiratory rates for a child 6 months to 1 year, 1 to 2 years, 3 to 6 years, 7 to 10 years, and 11 to 14 years of age?

24. What signs and symptoms would you look for when assessing an infant or a child for increased work of breathing?

25. Why is it harder to interpret chest sounds in a child?

26. Using the psychosocial stages of development described by Erikson, discuss how you would handle pediatric patients of various ages, as well as their parents or caregivers.

True/False

27. **T F** Parents should not be present when health-care providers are working with school-age children.

28. **T F** Infants and small children often have an intense need for their caregiver, so it is often helpful if the caregiver stays while you are providing care.

29. **T F** Never tell a child a procedure will be uncomfortable, because they will not allow you to perform the procedure once you've told them the truth.

30. **T F** When communicating with children, it is important to position yourself at or close to their eye level.

31. **T F** When treating older children and adolescents, it is important to encourage them to ask questions and participate in their own health care.

32. **T F** As a child's work of breathing increases, his or her activity level may decrease and feeding may become difficult.

33. **T F** In both infants and young children, the ratio of inspiration to expiration is fairly equal.

34. **T F** Signs of airway obstruction include prolonged expiratory phase and the use of abdominal muscles to facilitate expiration.

35. **T F** Cyanosis is an excellent indicator of hypoxemia; therefore, measurement of PaO_2 is rarely necessary in pediatric patients.

36. **T F** Accessory muscle use in children is manifested by retractions of supraclavicular, suprasternal, substernal, and intercostal muscles.

▨ Topic 3: Aerosol Delivery in the Pediatric Population ▨

37. What is the recommended mass median aerodynamic diameter (MMAD) for delivery of aerosol particles to the upper airway?

38. What are the indications for cool bland aerosol delivery?

39. State three indications for the administration of bland aerosol therapy.

40. What types of aerosol generator and patient application equipment can be used to administer bland aerosol therapy?

41. Give three examples of hazards/complications associated with bland aerosol therapy.

42. What factors influence aerosol particle deposition?

43. How should racemic epinephrine be delivered to children less than three years of age?

True/False

44. **T F**   Cool, wet mist may be irritating to children and can limit the time that the child tolerates an aerosol treatment.

45. **T F**   Nasal breathing results in a reduction in the deposition of aerosol particles to the lower airway.

46. **T F**   Contraindications to bland aerosol therapy include bronchoconstriction and a history of airway hyperresponsiveness.

47. **T F**   A small-volume nebulizer with a face mask can be used to deliver aerosolized medications to the upper airway in children less than three years of age.

48. **T F**   When delivering aerosolized medications to children three years of age and older, the RCP should use a small-volume nebulizer with a mouthpiece and an extension reservoir.

Topic 4: Follow-up to Alyssa Wilkinson

49. Alyssa presents with mild to moderate respiratory distress and stridor at rest. Describe the management of her condition.

50. Alyssa has been treated for the past 8 hours with nebulized racemic epinephrine at a dose of 0.5 ml of a 2.25% solution diluted to 3 ml volume with normal saline. The racemic epinephrine treatments are being ordered more frequently, and she is becoming exhausted and more distressed. What would you recommend?

51. Consider the following possibility: Alyssa comes to the emergency department with the following findings: sudden development of fever, severe sore throat, and difficulty swallowing. She is leaning forward and drooling and has an abnormal, muffled voice. How should she be treated?

POSTTEST

1. Which of the following is true regarding epiglottitis?

   a. It is most often caused by a virus.
   b. Drooling is common because of difficulty or pain of swallowing.
   c. Treatment includes racemic epinephrine.
   d. Low grade fever is commonly present.

2. The most common causative organism for laryngotracheobronchitis is:

   a. *Staphylococcus aureus*.
   b. parainfluenza virus.
   c. *Mycoplasma pneumoniae*.
   d. respiratory syncytial virus.

3. Which of the following is considered a contraindication to bland aerosol administration?

   a. laryngotracheobronchitis
   b. subglottic edema
   c. bronchoconstriction
   d. lung contusion

4. Problems associated with the nebulization of racemic epinephrine in children with croup include:

   a. a rebound or return of the original or worsened respiratory distress several hours after the treatment.
   b. the high cost and decreased availability of the drug.
   c. the awful taste of the drug, which makes it poorly tolerated by small children.
   d. a very slow onset of effect and potent cardiac stimulation.

5. Positive assessment of outcome following the administration of nebulized racemic epinephrine would include:

   I. improved vital signs.
   II. decreased stridor.
   III. decreased dyspnea.
   IV. improved oxygen saturation.

      a. IV only
      b. I and III only
      c. I, III, and IV only
      d. all of the above

6. Indication(s) for the administration of a water or isotonic or hypotonic saline aerosol include:

   I. brassy, croup-like cough.
   II. hoarseness following extubation.
   III. wheezing.
   IV. diagnosis of croup or laryngotracheobronchitis.

      a. I and II only
      b. III and IV only
      c. I, II, and IV only
      d. all of the above

7. The particle size for aerosol delivery to the upper airway should have a mass median aerodynamic diameter of greater than or equal to:

    a. one micron.
    b. two microns.
    c. three microns.
    d. five microns.

8. Patients diagnosed with croup can be safely treated at home with cool mist provided by a clean vaporizer when the:

    a. stridor occurs during exertion but not at rest.
    b. patient's voice is muffled and the fever is stable.
    c. stridor is present at rest but responds to nebulized racemic epinephrine.
    d. stridor is present on inspiration and expiration and intercostal retractions are present.

9. Which of the following is/are true concerning bacterial tracheitis?

    I.   The child often develops a high fever and has purulent tracheal secretions.
    II. Bacterial tracheitis is considered a life-threatening condition.
    III. Bacterial tracheitis is the most common form of croup.
    IV. Diagnosis is confirmed with cultures of blood and tracheal secretions.

        a. I and III only
        b. II and IV only
        c. I, II, and IV only
        d. all of the above

10. Techniques used to improve the outcome of an examination and/or treatment of an infant or small child include:

    I.   performing the most distressing components last.
    II. using distraction techniques.
    III. being honest with the child and the caregiver.
    IV. assessing the infant while on the caregiver's lap.

        a. II and III only
        b. I, III, and IV only
        c. I, II, and IV only
        d. all of the above

11. The standard dosage of nebulized racemic epinephrine for a child is:

    a. 0.2 to 0.5 ml of a 2.25% solution diluted to 3 ml volume with normal saline.
    b. 0.5 to 1.0 ml of a 2.25% solution diluted to 3 ml volume with normal saline.
    c. 0.5 to 1.0 ml of a 10% solution diluted to 3 ml volume with normal saline.
    d. 0.2 to 0.5 ml of a 1.0% solution diluted with 3 ml of atropine.

12. When trying to establish a professional rapport with older children or adolescents, you should:

    I.   avoid the use of condescending language.
    II. respect their privacy and the confidentiality of findings.
    III. examine, interview, and treat them only with a caregiver present.
    IV. provide them with feedback about their health status.

        a. I and II only
        b. III and IV only
        c. I, II, and IV only
        d. all of the above

13. Comparing the airway anatomic and physiologic differences between children and adults, children have:

    I.   smaller upper and lower airways.
    II. larger tongues in proportion to the size of the mouth.
    III. softer cartilage of the larynx.
    IV. higher normal respiratory rates.

        a. I, III, and IV only
        b. I and III only
        c. II and IV only
        d. all of the above

14. Classic croup most commonly affects children from the age range of:

        a. 6 months to 3 years.
        b. 3 years to 8 years.
        c. newborns up to 18 months.
        d. 6 years to 12 years.

15. Racemic epinephrine improves air flow in children with croup by:

        a. reducing the allergic inflammation.
        b. increasing blood flow to the swollen area to speed healing.
        c. reducing the subglottic edema through vasoconstriction.
        d. reducing the density of the inspired gas.

16. Characteristics of spasmodic croup include:

    I.   seasonal predilection and a viral prodrome.
    II. slowly progressive course with a constant low-grade fever.
    III. unknown etiology with a suspected allergic component.
    IV. onset often beginning during infancy and recurring until the age of four.

        a. I and IV only
        b. III and IV only
        c. I, II, and III only
        d. all of the above

17. Classic croup is known to be caused by:

    I. parainfluenza viruses.
    II. respiratory syncytial virus.
    III. *Mycoplasma pneumoniae.*
    IV. *Streptococcus pyogenes.*

       a. I and III only
       b. I and II only
       c. I, II, and III only
       d. all of the above

18. Initial therapy for epiglottitis focuses on:

    a. establishing an artificial airway.
    b. placing the child in a recumbent position.
    c. maintaining continuous cool mist therapy.
    d. administering nebulized antibiotics.

19. Infection control practices employed during bland aerosol therapy would include which of the following?

    I. implementing universal precautions for body fluid isolation
    II. observing all infection control guidelines posted for the patient
    III. disinfecting all equipment used between patients
    IV. providing frequent air exchanges to dilute the concentration of aerosol in the room

       a. I and II only
       b. II and III only
       c. III and IV only
       d. all of the above

20. According to the AARC Clinical Practice Guidelines for bland aerosol administration, hazards and complications of this therapy include:

    I. infection.
    II. wheezing or bronchospasm.
    III. overhydration.
    IV. patient discomfort.

       a. I and II only
       b. I and III only
       c. I, II, and III only
       d. all of the above

21. Monitoring of patients being treated for croup would include evaluation of:

    I. vital signs.
    II. accessory muscle use.
    III. changes in stridor.
    IV. changes in activity levels.

       a. I and II only
       b. I, II, and III only
       c. II, III, and IV only
       d. all of the above

22. Clinical situations indicating the need for intubation of a child being treated for croup would include:

    a. lack of response to therapy with noted exhaustion.
    b. spontaneous cough that fails to clear secretions.
    c. stridor at rest.
    d. mild to moderate distress after two hours in a croup tent.

23. When the diameter of the airway is decreased by half, the flow through the airway is decreased _____-fold.

    a. 2
    b. 4
    c. 16
    d. 32

24. Aerosol deposition is influenced by which of the following?

    I.   ventilatory pattern
    II. airway architecture
    III. particle size

        a. I and II only
        b. III only
        c. II and III only
        d. all of the above

25. A clinical presentation of a young child with a high fever, severe sore throat, drooling, muffled voice, and stridor best describes:

    a. epiglottitis.
    b. spasmodic croup.
    c. classic croup.
    d. laryngotracheobronchitis.

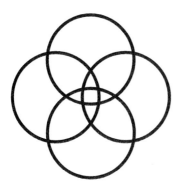

Noninvasive Monitoring

Resources

American Association for Respiratory Care: Clinical practice guideline: capnography/capnometry during mechanical ventilation, Resp Care 40:1321-1324, 1995.

American Association for Respiratory Care: Clinical practice guideline: pulse oximetry, Resp Care 36:1406-1409, 1991.

Barnes TA: Core textbook of respiratory care practice, ed 2, St. Louis, 1994, Mosby.

McPherson SP: Respiratory care equipment, ed 5, St. Louis, 1995, Mosby.

Pilbeam SP: Mechanical ventilation: physiologic and clinical applications, ed 2, St. Louis, 1992, Mosby.

Scanlan CL, Spearman CB, and Sheldon RL, editors: Egan's fundamentals of respiratory care, ed 6, St. Louis, 1995, Mosby.

Wilkins RL, Krider SJ, and Sheldon RL, editors: Clinical assessment in respiratory care, ed 3, St. Louis, 1995, Mosby.

Topic 1: Electrocardiography

1. On the electrocardiogram pictured below, label the P and T waves and the QRS complex.

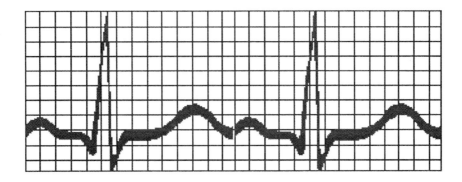

2. Describe the major electrical events of the cardiac cycle seen on an electrocardiogram.

3. What does the P-R interval represent, and what is its normal length of time?

4. What does the S-T segment represent, and what is its normal value?

5. What does the Q-T segment represent, and what is the significance of a prolonged Q-T segment?

True/False

6. **T F**   The SA node is the primary pacemaker of the heart.

7. **T F**   The inherent rate of the SA node is 60 to 100 beats per minute.

8. **T F**   The inherent rate of the AV node is 40 to 60 beats per minute.

9. **T F**   The QRS duration normally measures 0.04 to 0.10 seconds.

10. **T F**   On an electrocardiograph tracing, each one-millimeter box represents 0.04 seconds.

11. **T F**   Atrial depolarization is represented by the R wave.

12. **T F**   When the rhythm is regular, heart rate can be determined by counting the number of large squares (5 small boxes) between two R waves and dividing by 300.

13. **T F**   A normal P-R interval is 0.04 to 0.10 second.

14. **T F**   The normal Q wave is less than 25% of the amplitude of the R wave.

15. **T F**   The primary role of the AV node is to delay, and then relay, the SA nodal impulses to the ventricles.

Matching

Match the following diagrams (Figures 7-2a–h) to the proper description.

16. _____   normal sinus rhythm

17. _____   sinus bradycardia

18. _____   atrial fibrillation

19. _____   atrial flutter

20. _____   ventricular tachycardia

21. _____   sinus rhythm with PVC

22. _____   sinus tachycardia

23. _____   asystole

A

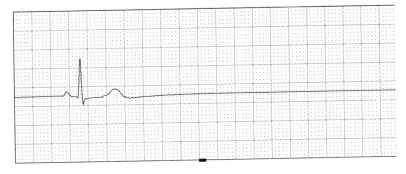

B

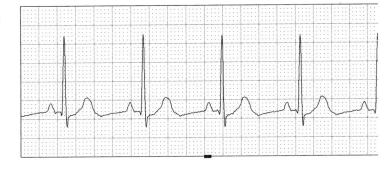

C

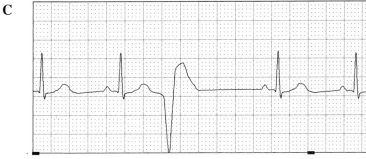

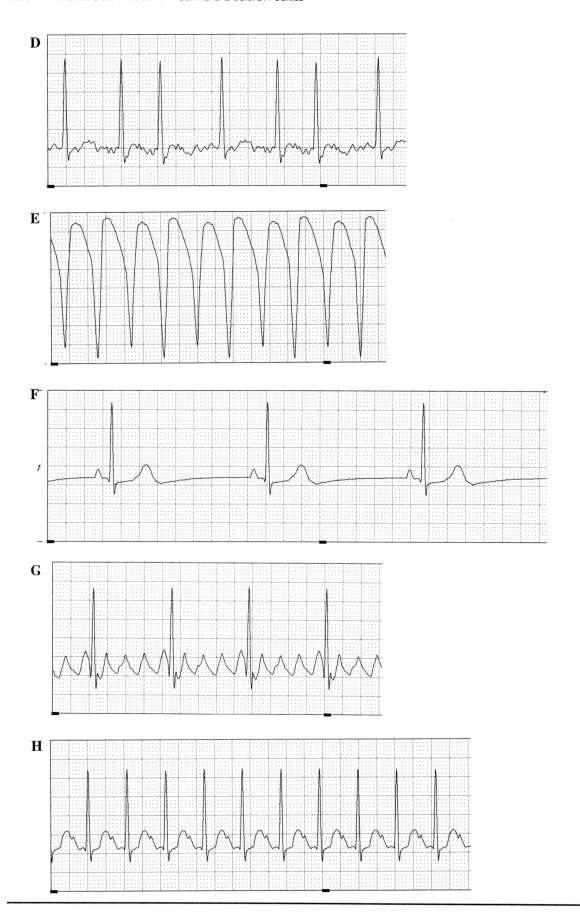

Figures 7-2a–h Courtesy of SpaceLabs Medical, Inc., Redmond, Washington.

Topic 2: Pulse Oximetry

24. Describe the principles of operation for the pulse oximeter.

25. Why is it important to consider the oxyhemoglobin dissociation curve when you are trying to make an assessment of a patient's oxygenation using a saturation reading from a pulse oximeter?

26. State the indications for use of a pulse oximeter.

27. Write the contraindications for pulse oximetry.

28. Discuss the factors that can limit the accuracy, precision, or performance of the pulse oximeter.

29. Describe how to validate pulse oximeter readings in the clinical setting.

True/False

30. **T F**   The presence of carboxyhemoglobin can result in an underestimation of arterial oxyhemoglobin saturation.

31. **T F**   Direct sunlight shining on the patient probe can cause the SpO_2 reading to be higher than actual oxyhemoglobin saturation.

32. **T F**   The use of pulse oximetry is indicated during interventions such as bronchoscopy, where desaturation episodes are likely to occur.

33. **T F**   Conditions such as hypovolemia, hypotension, and hypothermia may cause a low pulse signal, and therefore, result in a saturation reading by pulse oximetry that will not necessarily correlate with directly measured arterial values.

34. **T F**   Hyperbilirubinemia in infants has been shown to decrease the accuracy of pulse oximetry measurement of oxyhemoglobin saturation.

35. **T F**   Pulse oximeters are generally capable of measuring oxyhemoglobin saturation above 60% with an accuracy of ± 4%.

36. **T F**   In all clinical circumstances, SpO_2 readings reflect the patient's clinical condition as accurately as direct measurement of arterial oxyhemoglobin saturation.

37. **T F**   To validate a SpO_2 reading, the respiratory care practitioner should initially compare the reading with that of a directly measured oxyhemoglobin saturation.

38. **T F**   The presence of an ongoing need to measure pH, $PaCO_2$, and total hemoglobin is a relative contraindication to pulse oximetry.

39. **T F**   Pulse oximetry detects low and high oxyhemoglobin saturations with the same accuracy.

▰▰ Topic 3: Capnography ▰▰▰▰▰▰▰▰▰▰▰▰▰▰▰▰▰▰▰▰▰▰▰▰

40. Define the terms *capnometry* and *capnography*.

41. How is exhaled carbon dioxide measured at the bedside?

42. Exhaled gases for capnographic analysis are collected in two ways. What are the two methods of collection, and how do they differ?

43. List two advantages for each of the two methods of capnographic analysis described in the answer to question 42.

44. Describe what you would look for when evaluating a patient's CO_2 waveform.

45. What is the normal gradient between the arterial carbon dioxide level and the exhaled end-tidal carbon dioxide level [P(a-et)CO_2]?

46. What effect does the relationship between ventilation and perfusion of the lungs have on end-tidal carbon dioxide levels?

47. Describe the clinical uses for capnography.

48. Explain the role capnography plays during endotracheal intubation of a patient.

True/False

49. **T F** Monitoring with capnography is considered a standard of care during anesthesia.

50. **T F** Contamination of the capnography monitor or sampling system by secretions or condensate can lead to unreliable results.

51. **T F** As dead-space volume increases, so will the difference between $PEtCO_2$ and $PaCO_2$.

52. **T F** The gradient between $PaCO_2$ and $PEtCO_2$ is normally 5 to 10 mm Hg.

53. **T F** End-tidal carbon dioxide levels vary with changes in carbon dioxide production, carbon dioxide delivery to the lungs, and changes in alveolar ventilation.

54. **T F** Sidestream capnographs cannot be used with nonintubated patients; mainstream capnographs must be used.

55. **T F** $PEtCO_2$ levels of greater than 15 mm Hg have been associated with patients likely to be resuscitated, whereas values of less than 15 mm Hg have been associated with patients who cannot be resuscitated.

56. **T F** $PEtCO_2$ is usually considerably lower than the $PaCO_2$ in pulmonary hypoperfusion states.

57. **T F** Capnography is useful in determining correct endotracheal tube placement, detecting tubing disconnection during mechanical ventilation, and monitoring systemic perfusion during cardiopulmonary resuscitation.

58. **T F** The normal $PEtCO_2$ is between 4.5% and 5.5% of exhaled gas.

Matching

Match the diagrams below (Figures 7-3a–g) to the proper type of breathing pattern or clinical condition.

59. _____ hyperventilation (single waveform)

60. _____ hyperventilation following a period of normal ventilation

61. _____ hypoventilation (single waveform)

62. _____ hypoventilation following a period of normal ventilation

63. _____ leak in system

64. _____ patient fighting the ventilator

65. _____ emphysema

A

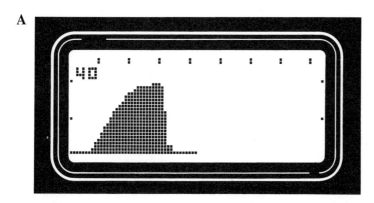

B

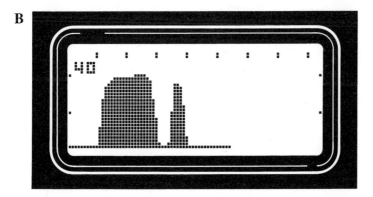

C

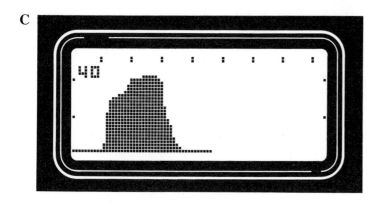

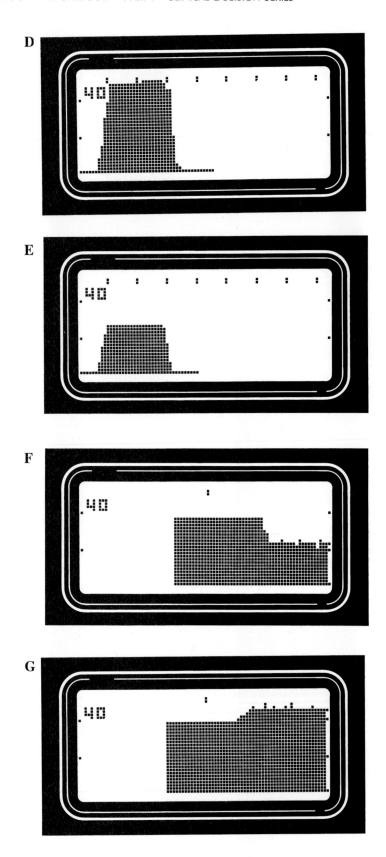

Figures 7-3a–g Courtesy of Ohmeda, Inc., Louisville, Colorado.

■ Topic 4: Follow-up to Beatrice Reilly ▬▬▬▬▬▬▬

Refer to the therapist-driven protocol on page 210 to complete the following.

66. Beatrice Reilly is still in the emergency department and she has received activated charcoal through her nasogastric tube and naloxone by IV. She is intubated and being monitored by ECG, pulse oximeter, and capnograph. During an injection of 50 mEq of sodium bicarbonate by IV, she had a tonic-clonic seizure that lasted at least 30 seconds. What would you expect to see on the capnograph?

67. Ms. Reilly is transferred to the intensive care unit for observation and monitoring. She remains intubated on a 30% T-piece. Four hours after admission to the ICU, the ECG monitor reveals a prolonged PR interval and widened QRS. In addition, she is experiencing episodes of desaturation and her capnogram is shown in Figure 7-3g on the previous page. What would you recommend?

68. Twenty-four hours after admission to the ICU, the patient remains on a 30% oxygen blow-by set-up. She continues to have sinus tachycardia with occasional premature ventricular contractions. She is also experiencing seizures with desaturations noted by pulse oximetry. Is she still a candidate for continuous pulse oximetry monitoring? Explain your reasoning.

69. Twenty-four hours after admission to the ICU, Ms. Reilly's condition deteriorates. Pulse oximetry reveals significant desaturation, her respiratory rate, blood pressure, and heart rate are all elevated, and she is agitated. Auscultation reveals rhonchi bilaterally, she requires frequent suctioning for pale yellow secretions, and her chest x-ray reveals patchy infiltrates. What is a likely cause of her clinical signs? What would you recommend?

70. Ms. Reilly requires continuous mechanical ventilatory support. Her vital signs stabilize, saturation levels return to 95%, and the capnograph demonstrates stable CO_2 readings. One hour later, you look at the capnograph and see the tracing below. What does this tracing indicate?

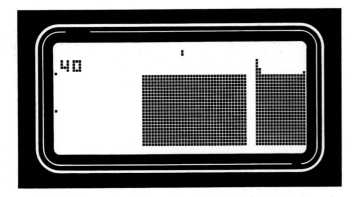

Trend.

Figure 7-4 Courtesy of Ohmeda, Inc., Louisville, Colorado.

1. The gradient between $PaCO_2$ and $PEtCO_2$ is usually:

   a. less than 5 mm Hg.
   b. 5 to 10 mm Hg.
   c. 10 to 15 mm Hg.
   d. greater than 25 mm Hg.

2. Most bedside capnographs measure CO_2 by:

   a. mass spectrometry.
   b. infrared absorption.
   c. Raman scattering.
   d. plethysmography.

3. The P wave on an electrocardiogram represents:

   a. atrial repolarization.
   b. ventricular depolarization.
   c. atrial depolarization.
   d. the firing of the AV node.

4. To validate pulse oximeter readings, the respiratory care practitioner should:

   a. complete a high/low calibration before use on each patient.
   b. assess agreement between SpO_2 and directly measured SaO_2.
   c. clean the probe with alcohol before each use.
   d. allow the equipment to self-calibrate.

5. Factors that may affect pulse oximeter readings include:

   I.   low perfusion states.
   II. hyperbilirubinemia.
   III. abnormal hemoglobin.
   IV. intravascular dyes.

      a. II and IV only
      b. I and III only
      c. I, III, and IV only
      d. all of the above

6. Which of the following are true concerning the QRS complex?

   I.   The QRS represents ventricular depolarization.
   II. The QRS normally measures 0.04 to 0.10 seconds in adults.
   III. The QRS represents ventricular repolarization.
   IV. The QRS has a normal amplitude of 5 mm.

      a. I and II only
      b. III and IV only
      c. I, II, and IV only
      d. all of the above

7. When evaluating an electrocardiogram, if you count the number of large squares (5 small boxes) between two R waves and divide 300 by that number, you will be able to determine the:

   a. rhythm.
   b. rate.
   c. number of escape beats.
   d. P-R interval.

8. The normal $PEtCO_2$ is between _____% and _____% in exhaled gas.

   a. 4.5, 5.5
   b. 2, 10
   c. 25, 35
   d. 11.2, 15.2

9. Which of the following conditions cause an increase in CO_2 production and delivery to the lungs and, therefore, can cause an increased $PEtCO_2$ when there is no compensation through alveolar ventilation?

   I.   sepsis
   II. fever
   III. seizures
   IV. hypothermia

      a. I and II only
      b. II, III, and IV only
      c. I, II, and III only
      d. all of the above

10. Causes of decreased $PEtCO_2$ values include:

   I.   ventilator disconnection.
   II. endotracheal tube cuff leaks.
   III. esophageal intubation.
   IV. hyperventilation.

      a. II and IV only
      b. I, III, and IV only
      c. I, II, and IV only
      d. all of the above

11. Phase II of the capnogram pictured below represents:

    a. anatomic deadspace gas.
    b. alveolar gas mixing with deadspace gas.
    c. gas from alveolar emptying.
    d. an area of high $\dot{V}/\dot{Q}$.

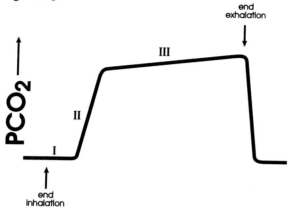

Figure 7-5 From Barnes TA: Core textbook of respiratory care practice, ed 2, St. Louis, 1994, Mosby.

12. The technology incorporated in pulse oximetry includes:

    I.   Raman scattering.
    II. spectrophotometry.
    III. photoplethysmography.
    IV. mass spectrometry.

        a. I and II only
        b. III and IV only
        c. II, III, and IV only
        d. II and III only

13. Which of the following conditions have the potential to cause a falsely high pulse oximeter reading?

    I.   low perfusion states
    II. direct sunlight on the probe
    III. presence of carboxyhemoglobin
    IV. presence of methemoglobin

        a. I and II only
        b. I and IV only
        c. II, III, and IV only
        d. all of the above

14. Atrial flutter is identified by its classic:

    a. sawtooth pattern.
    b. rounded P waves.
    c. inverted QRS complex.
    d. escape beats.

15. The P-R interval represents:

    a. ventricular depolarization.
    b. the length of time required for the electrical stimulus to spread through the atria and to pass through the AV junction.
    c. the relative refractory period during which ventricles are at risk for dysrhythmia.
    d. early repolarization of the right and left ventricles.

16. Advantages of mainstream capnography include:

    I.   lack of sample flow, which reduces exhaled tidal volume measurements.
    II. real-time readings.
    III. very fast response times.
    IV. its ability to be used on nonintubated patients.

        a. I and II only
        b. II and III only
        c. I, II, and III only
        d. all of the above

17. Atrial fibrillation is characterized by a(n):

    I.   irregular rhythm.
    II. atrial rate greater than 400.
    III. absence of P waves.
    IV. QRS less than 0.10.

        a. I and III only
        b. I and II only
        c. II, III, and IV only
        d. all of the above

18. The use of a slow capnogram will help to identify CO_2 rebreathing by demonstrating:

    a. a $PEtCO_2$ level that does not return to baseline.
    b. a slow rise of $PEtCO_2$ at phase II.
    c. $PEtCO_2$ levels that remain high.
    d. a $PEtCO_2$ level that rises slowly over time.

19. Which of the following arrhythmias is most life-threatening?

    a. atrial fibrillation
    b. ventricular fibrillation
    c. atrial flutter
    d. sinus tachycardia

20. The alveolar level of CO_2 is determined by the:

    I.   rate of metabolism and the production of CO_2.
    II. removal of CO_2 from the lungs through ventilation.
    III. rate of perfusion of blood through the lungs.

        a. I and II only
        b. I and III only
        c. II and III only
        d. all of the above

21. Supraventricular tachycardia is characterized by a:

    I.   regular rhythm.
    II. rate of 160 to 250.
    III. QRS less than 0.10.
    IV. P-R segment greater than 2.0.

        a. I and III only
        b. I, II, and III only
        c. II, III, and IV only
        d. all of the above

22. Causes of decreased alveolar ventilation that may result in an increased $PEtCO_2$ include:

    I.   COPD.
    II. respiratory center depression.
    III. muscular weakness/paralysis.
    IV. alveolar hypoventilation.

        a. I and IV only
        b. I, II, and III only
        c. II, III, and IV only
        d. all of the above

23. Abnormalities in atrial depolarization can result in:

    I.   sinus tachycardia.
    II. sinus bradycardia.
    III. atrial fibrillation.
    IV. atrial flutter.

        a. I and II only
        b. II and III only
        c. III and IV only
        d. all of the above

24. The dominant pacemaker of the heart is the:

        a. AV node.
        b. SA node
        c. bundle of His.
        d. Purkinje system.

25. $PEtCO_2$ levels that remain near zero are associated with:

        a. esophageal intubation.
        b. decreased cardiac output.
        c. injection of sodium bicarbonate.
        d. air embolism.

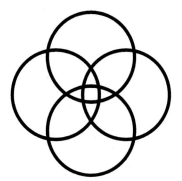

Mechanical Ventilation

Resources

Des Jardins T and Burton GG: Clinical manifestations and assessment of respiratory disease, ed 3, St. Louis, 1995, Mosby.

McCance KL and Huether SE: Pathophysiology: the biologic basis for disease in adults and children, ed 2, St. Louis, 1994, Mosby.

Pilbeam SP: Mechanical ventilation: physiologic and clinical applications, ed 2, St. Louis, 1992, Mosby.

Scanlan CL, Spearman CB, and Sheldon RL, editors: Egan's fundamentals of respiratory care, ed 6, St. Louis, 1995, Mosby.

Topic 1: Mechanical Ventilation

1. Differentiate between full ventilatory support and partial ventilatory support, and give one example describing when each is indicated.

2. Describe each of the following: CMV, A/C, SIMV, PSV, PCV, MMV, APRV, and BiPAP®.

3. What are the indications for mechanical ventilation?

4. List the values for the following parameters that indicate the need for ventilatory support:

Tidal volume: _____ ml/kg

Vital capacity: _____ ml/kg

Respiratory rate: _____ breaths/min

Maximum inspiratory pressure: _____ cm H_2O

$PaCO_2$: _____ mm Hg

PaO_2: _____ mm Hg (room air), _____ mm Hg (oxygen)

Arterial/alveolar PO_2 ratio (PaO_2/PAO_2): _____

5. List the parameters used when setting the following ventilator alarms: high minute ventilation, low minute ventilation, high tidal volume, low tidal volume, high inspiratory pressure limit, low inspiratory pressure, low PEEP/CPAP, and FIO_2.

6. Describe the initial assessment of a patient on mechanical ventilation.

7. What are the goals of mechanical ventilatory support?

8. Describe how the initial tidal volume setting is determined for volume-cycled ventilation of the adult patient.

9. Describe how the target minute ventilation is determined when instituting mechanical ventilation for an adult patient.

10. When initiating volume-cycled mechanical ventilation on an adult patient, explain how you would determine an appropriate flowrate.

11. What are the physiologic goals of mechanical ventilation?

12. You are caring for a patient on volume-cycled ventilation, and the $PaCO_2$ is rising. Explain how you would adjust the ventilatory parameters to maintain adequate ventilation at safe ventilating pressures.

13. For patients requiring mechanical ventilation, how is oxygenation adjusted?

14. What are the indications for providing sigh breaths? At what volume and rate are they set during mechanical ventilatory support of a patient?

15. Calculate the static compliance and airway resistance for a patient on the following settings, and determine if the values are increased, decreased, or normal for a mechanically ventilated patient: CMV rate: 15, FIO_2: 45%, PEEP: 5 cm H_2O, peak inspiratory pressure: 37 cm H_2O, plateau pressure: 35 cm H_2O, delivered tidal volume: 500 ml, and flowrate: 60 L/minute.

16. Briefly discuss the care and assessment of the endotracheal tube following intubation.

True/False

17. **T F**   The best available indicators for inadequate muscle strength are $PaCO_2$ and pH.

18. **T F**   A maximum inspiratory pressure of less than 20 cm H_2O indicates the need for ventilatory support.

19. **T F**   A rapid rate of breathing is a sign of increased work of breathing.

20. **T F** PSV_{max} cannot be used to provide full ventilatory support.

21. **T F**   To avoid alveolar overdistention, it is recommended that respiratory care practitioners use lower tidal volumes and pressures when ventilating patients.

22. **T F**   When patients' static compliance is less than 25 ml/cm H_2O, their work of breathing is increased.

23. **T F**   Normal airway resistance with an endotracheal tube in place is 6 to 18 cm H_2O/L/second.

24. **T F**   High-pressure alarms are usually set 10 cm H_2O above the average peak airway pressure when using volume-cycled mechanical ventilation.

25. **T F**   Inappropriately applied mechanical ventilation can increase the patient's work of breathing and increase oxygen consumption.

26. **T F**   The peak inspiratory flowrate should be set at a low value (less than 50 L/min) to avoid auto-PEEP with mechanical ventilation.

Matching

Match the tidal volume and frequency on the right to the patient type on the left. Tidal volume and frequency descriptions can be used more than once.

27. _____ adult with normal lungs

28. _____ adult with chronic obstructive pulmonary disease

29. _____ adult with ARDS

30. _____ child 8 to 16 years of age

31. _____ adult with restrictive lung disease

A. tidal volume of 12 to 15 ml/kg and a rate of 8 to 12

B. tidal volume of 10 ml/kg or less and a rate of 12 to 20

C. tidal volume of 10 to 12 ml/kg and a rate of 8 to 10

D. tidal volume of 8 to 10 ml/kg and a rate of 20 to 30

▬ Topic 2: PEEP Therapy ▬

32. What are the indications for PEEP therapy?

33. What are the contraindications to PEEP therapy?

34. What are the beneficial physiologic effects of PEEP?

35. What are the detrimental physiologic effects of PEEP?

36. Explain how PEEP is administered and monitored.

True/False

37. **T F** PEEP improves oxygenation by increasing the FRC and decreasing physiologic shunting.

38. **T F** Underwater columns, spring-loaded diaphragms or disks, and electromechanical valves can all be used to generate PEEP.

39. **T F** A hazard of PEEP therapy is decreased intracranial pressure.

40. **T F** CPAP can be applied to the airway by means of nasal prongs, face mask, nasal mask, or endotracheal tube.

41. **T F** When weaning a patient from PEEP, if the PaO_2 falls more than 20% along with an increase in shunt, the PEEP should be returned to the previous level.

▬ Topic 3: Pulmonary Edema/Myocardial Infarction/Congestive Heart Failure ▬

42. Define pulmonary edema.

43. What is the etiology of pulmonary edema?

44. Describe the differences seen in the chest radiograph of cardiogenic pulmonary edema versus noncardiogenic pulmonary edema.

45. Describe the classic clinical presentation of pulmonary edema.

46. Are supplemental oxygen therapy and hyperinflation techniques beneficial in cases of pulmonary edema?

47. What is a myocardial infarction?

48. Describe the clinical manifestations of a myocardial infarction.

49. What are the functional changes associated with myocardial infarction?

50. Describe some of the complications associated with myocardial infarction.

51. What is congestive heart failure?

True/False

52. **T F** The most common complication of acute myocardial infarction is dysrhythmia.

53. **T F** Cardiac cells can withstand ischemic conditions for about 20 minutes before cellular death occurs.

54. **T F** Treatment of pulmonary edema includes the use of diuretic agents to promote fluid excretion.

55. **T F** Morphine sulfate is used to increase afterload and venous pooling in the treatment of pulmonary edema.

56. **T F** Severe pulmonary edema can result in acute ventilatory failure with hypoxemia.

57. **T F** The severity of functional impairment following a myocardial infarction depends on the size of the lesion and the site of the infarction.

58. **T F** Hemodynamic indices of cardiogenic pulmonary edema include decreases in cardiac output, right atrial pressure, mean pulmonary artery pressure, and pulmonary wedge pressure.

59. **T F** The diagnosis of acute myocardial infarction is confirmed using ECG, serial enzyme results, radionucleotide imaging, and physical examination.

60. **T F** Causes of pulmonary edema in which the exact mechanism is not known include encephalitis, head trauma, and metal poisoning.

61. **T F** Myocardial infarction occurs exclusively in the posterior region of the heart.

Topic 4: Follow-up to Mrs. Gleason

Refer to the therapist-driven protocol on page 211 to complete the following.

62. Mrs. Gleason is on a ventilator with the following settings: SIMV rate 10, tidal volume 750 ml, FIO_2 0.40, PEEP +3 cm H_2O. Her ABG results are pH 7.37, $PaCO_2$ 44, HCO_3 25, PaO_2 41, and SaO_2 75%. What changes in the ventilator settings would you make?

63. Mrs. Gleason is on a ventilator with the following settings: SIMV rate 10, tidal volume 750 ml, FIO_2 0.40, PEEP +3 cm H_2O. Her spontaneous rate is zero. Her ABG results are pH 7.22, $PaCO_2$ 63, HCO_3 25, PaO_2 101, and SaO_2 98%. What changes in the ventilator settings would you make?

64. Mrs. Gleason is on a ventilator with the following settings: PC 25 cm H_2O, rate 10, FIO_2 0.40, PEEP +3 cm H_2O. Her ABG results are pH 7.32, $PaCO_2$ 56, HCO_3 27, PaO_2 108, and SaO_2 96%. What changes in the ventilator settings would you make?

65. Mrs. Gleason is on a ventilator with the following settings: PSV 25 cm H_2O, FIO_2 0.40, and PEEP +3 cm H_2O. Her vital signs are stable, and she has a respiratory rate of 18. Breath sounds are clear except for inspiratory crackles at the bases. Her ABG results are pH 7.45, $PaCO_2$ 32, HCO_3 21, PaO_2 82, and SaO_2 94%. What changes in the ventilator settings would you make?

66. Twenty-four hours after initiation of mechanical ventilation, Mrs. Gleason has responded well to therapy. Her breath sounds are clear with fine crackles at the bases, and she is alert and writing messages frequently to the RCP and nurse. She is on PSV of 20 cm H_2O, FIO_2 of 0.35, and PEEP of +3 cm H_2O. Her respiratory rate is 16, and her SpO_2 is 96%. Weaning parameters are as follows: maximum inspiratory force -40 cm H_2O, vital capacity 1800 ml, minute volume 7.2 L, $\dot{Q}s/\dot{Q}t$ 9%, ABG and vital signs stable. What would you recommend?

POSTTEST

1. A patient is breathing spontaneously while pressure above atmospheric is maintained at the airway opening throughout the breathing cycle. This best describes:

   a. synchronized intermittent mandatory ventilation.
   b. pressure control ventilation.
   c. continuous positive airway pressure.
   d. pressure support.

2. When using a pressure-targeted mode of ventilation, an increase in lung compliance will most likely result in a/an:

   a. increase in delivered tidal volume.
   b. decrease in delivered tidal volume.
   c. altered machine sensitivity.
   d. increase in respiratory rate.

3. A patient is on pressure control ventilation with an FIO_2 of 0.80 and has a PaO_2 of 49 mm Hg and an SaO_2 of 86%. PEEP was titrated to +10 cm H_2O, with a resulting increase in PaO_2 to 102 mm Hg. Which of the following best explains these results?

   a. leftward shift of the oxyhemoglobin curve
   b. decreased physiologic shunting
   c. decreased compliance of the lungs
   d. increased alveolar ventilation

4. A patient on volume-targeted mechanical ventilation is retaining CO_2. What change in ventilator settings will correct the problem and decrease deadspace ventilation per minute?

   a. increasing the rate
   b. decreasing the rate
   c. increasing the tidal volume
   d. decreasing the tidal volume

5. Which of the following factors affect airway resistance?

   I. size, shape, and caliber of the airways
   II. pattern of gas flow
   III. characteristics of the gas being breathed

   a. I only
   b. I and II only
   c. II and III only
   d. all of the above

6. Which of the following criteria are considered to be indications of acute respiratory failure and the need for mechanical ventilatory support?

    I.   maximum inspiratory pressure of -50 to -100 cm H_2O
    II. tidal volume less than 5 ml/kg
    III. VD/VT greater than 0.6
    IV. arterial/alveolar PO_2 of 0.75

       a. I and II only
       b. III and IV only
       c. II and III only
       d. all of the above

7. A patient requires mechanical ventilation because of a drug overdose that has resulted in her inability to maintain an airway; she requires ventilatory support because of an irregular breathing pattern. Which of the following ventilatory modes would you suggest for this patient?

    a. continuous positive airway pressure
    b. assist/control
    c. pressure support
    d. flow-by

8. Which of the following ventilatory modes is best described as "pressure-limited assisted ventilation designed to augment a spontaneously generated breath"?

    a. continuous positive airway pressure
    b. assist/control ventilation
    c. pressure support
    d. synchronized intermittent mandatory ventilation

9. Your patient is being ventilated with a volume-limited mode. You notice the peak airway pressure has suddenly increased from 35 cm H_2O to 50 cm H_2O and is triggering the alarm. Which of the following factors are possible causes of this condition?

    I.   a large leak in the system
    II. kinked ventilator tubing
    III. patient-ventilator asynchrony
    IV. airway secretions or plugs

       a. I, II, and III only
       b. II, III, and IV only
       c. I, II, and IV only
       d. all of the above

10. Your patient is being ventilated on the following settings: SIMV rate of 8, tidal volume of 800 ml, FIO_2 of 0.40, and + 10 cm H_2O of PEEP. You note a peak airway pressure of 35 cm H_2O for each machine breath, an average total respiratory rate of 14 breaths per minute, and a total minute ventilation of 8 liters. Which of the following alarm settings are appropriate?

    I.   low minute ventilation of 3 liters
    II. high pressure limit of 45 cm H_2O
    III. FIO_2 at 0.35 and 0.45
    IV. high respiratory rate at 40

    a. II and IV only
    b. II and III only
    c. I, II, and III only
    d. all of the above

11. A patient being mechanically ventilated in the pressure control mode and monitored in the intensive care unit has an episode of significant desaturation and bradycardia. The low inspiratory pressure and exhaled tidal volume alarms are sounding. You would:

    a. check the ventilator tubing and humidifier for leaks.
    b. draw an arterial blood gas immediately.
    c. disconnect the patient and ventilate with a manual resuscitator.
    d. change the patient from pressure control ventilation to assist/control ventilation.

12. Detrimental effects of PEEP therapy include all of the following *except*:

    a. decreased shunt fraction.
    b. increased pulmonary vascular resistance.
    c. increased intracranial pressure.
    d. decreased venous return.

13. Causes of cardiogenic pulmonary edema include:

    I.   adult respiratory distress syndrome.
    II. left ventricular failure.
    III. systemic hypertension.
    IV. myocardial infarction.

    a. I and II only
    b. I and IV only
    c. II, III, and IV only
    d. I, II, and IV only

14. The I:E ratio alarm is activated, indicating that the I:E ratio has approached 1:1. Which adjustment would correct this situation?

    a. increasing the peak flow
    b. adding an inspiratory hold
    c. increasing the respiratory rate
    d. decreasing the peak flow

15. A patient is being ventilated at a rate of 10 breaths per minute and at a tidal volume of 600 ml. His $PaCO_2$ on these settings is 50 mm Hg. What tidal volume is needed to bring the patient's $PaCO_2$ to 40 mm Hg?

    a. 500 ml
    b. 550 ml
    c. 650 ml
    d. 750 ml

16. Clinical manifestations of cardiogenic pulmonary edema include:

    I. increased shunting.
    II. decreased oxygen delivery.
    III. decreased mixed venous saturation.
    IV. decreased functional residual capacity.

        a. I and II only
        b. II and III only
        c. I, II, and III only
        d. all of the above

17. A patient is being ventilated with the following settings: SIMV rate of 12, tidal volume: 600 ml, FIO_2: 0.45, PEEP: +10 cm H_2O. He becomes disconnected from the ventilator. Which of the following alarms would be activated?

    I. high pressure limit
    II. high minute ventilation
    III. low tidal volume
    IV. low PEEP/CPAP

        a. I and III only
        b. I and II only
        c. III and IV only
        d. II and III only

18. A patient is being ventilated with a pressure-limited mode of ventilation and has arterial blood gas values indicating a respiratory acidosis. The recommended action is to:

    a. increase the pressure limit.
    b. decrease the pressure limit.
    c. change to a volume-targeted mode.
    d. switch to a square wave flow pattern.

19. What FIO_2 is needed to raise a patient's PaO_2 from 60 mm Hg to 80 mm Hg when on an FIO_2 of 0.30?

    a. 0.50
    b. 0.40
    c. 0.60
    d. 0.80

20. The management of pulmonary edema can include:

    I. supplemental oxygen.
    II. morphine sulfate.
    III. diuretic therapy.
    IV. CPAP therapy.

        a. I and II only
        b. I and III only
        c. I, II, and IV only
        d. all of the above

21. Functional impairment resulting from myocardial infarction includes:

    I. increased cardiac contractility.
    II. decreased ejection fraction.
    III. sinoatrial node malfunction.
    IV. increased stroke volume.

        a. I and III only
        b. II and III only
        c. II, III, and IV only
        d. all of the above

22. Goals of mechanical ventilation can include:

    I. correction of acute respiratory acidosis.
    II. reduction of intracranial pressure.
    III. decrease in myocardial oxygen consumption.
    IV. relief of respiratory distress.

        a. I and IV only
        b. I, II, and III only
        c. II, III, and IV only
        d. all of the above

23. In which of the following clinical situations is pressure support ventilation appropriate?

    I. as a method of ventilator weaning
    II. to reduce the work of breathing through an endotracheal tube
    III. for a patient with periods of apnea requiring ventilation
    IV. for long-term support of a paralyzed patient

        a. I and II only
        b. II and III only
        c. I only
        d. all of the above

24. Your patient has a peak inspiratory pressure of 35 cm H_2O, tidal volume of 500 ml, PEEP of +5 cm H_2O, plateau pressure of 25 cm H_2O, and a respiratory rate of 15. His static compliance is _____ ml/cm H_2O.

    a. 14
    b. 17
    c. 20
    d. 25

25. The best value with which to determine the adequacy of ventilation is:

   a. $PaCO_2$.
   b. vital capacity.
   c. VD/VT.
   d. $\dot{Q}s/\dot{Q}t$.

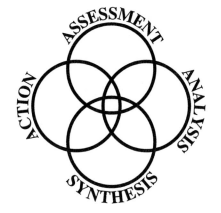

Part II

Answers to Clinical Decision Series

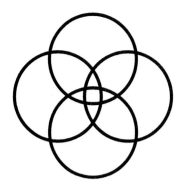

Answers to Clinical Decision Series

Introductory Unit: Introduction to Clinical Decision Making

Topic: Aspects of Clinical Decision Making

1. CPGs are systematically developed statements designed to assist clinicians in providing appropriate and targeted care for their patients. Respiratory care guidelines follow a standard format which includes a description or definition of the procedure; the setting for performance; indications, contraindications, hazards/complications of the procedure; limitations of the procedure or device; assessment of need and of outcome; resources required; procedure monitoring; frequency determination; infection control requirements; and supporting references.

2. The American Association for Respiratory Care supported the development of CPGs for Respiratory Care to improve the consistency, appropriateness, and patient outcomes of respiratory care throughout the country. CPG development provides a broad framework from which specific institutional policies, procedures, and protocols can be generated.

3. The AARC Clinical Practice Guidelines were developed through an initiative that began in 1990 with the development of the Steering Committee. The Steering Committee organized and continues to organize and oversee working committees charged with specific guideline development. The foundation of the process is a thorough literature review coupled with surveys of current practice and committee member expertise. CPG drafts developed by the working committees are reviewed by consultants, peers, experts, and the Steering Committee. Once appropriate revisions are made the CPG is published and widely distributed.

4. CPGs are used to support respiratory care education and research. They are used in the clinical setting to develop policies, procedures, protocols, critical pathways, and consultation programs.

5. TDPs were defined by Judy Tietsort, RN, RRT and George Burton, MD, as "patient care plans which are initiated and implemented by credentialed respiratory care workers." They are created with the input of physicians and other health care professionals and are approved for use by the medical staff and governing body of the institution. When properly designed and implemented, the respiratory care professional has the authority and responsibility to evaluate the patient, initiate care, and modify/discontinue/re-start care based on patient need within scope of the protocol.

6. TDPs are also called patient-driven protocols and respiratory care plans.

7. TDPs have been developed for a number of reasons. The development and increasing use of TDPs has been fueled in part by the demands of an ever-changing health-care system including restructuring, cost containment, and changes in the allocation of patient care. Studies have shown respiratory care providers can allocate respiratory care services better than other health-care providers. The development of CPGs has helped define the indications for respiratory care modalities and has provided a firm foundation for the development of credible institutional TDPs.

8. The advantages TDPs offer when compared to traditional physician ordered therapy include the following: (1) allocation of respiratory services (less over-ordering and under-ordering of respiratory care) is improved, (2) patient assessment and adjustment of care based in response to changes in

157

patient condition is more timely, (3) respiratory care practitioners become actively involved in achieving patient centered goals, (4) practitioners practice what they learned in school and are less frustrated compared to practitioners performing rigid tasks, (5) practitioners are continually learning through case challenges and peer review, (6) fewer "nuisance calls" to physicians.

9. The AARC Clinical Practice Guidelines can be used as a standardized foundation for the development of individualized institutional TDPs.

10. Clinical decision making skills are the cornerstone of patient care based on TDPs. To be valuable and respected members of health care teams, respiratory care practitioners must be skilled clinical decision makers.

11. One model of clinical decision making includes four steps: assessment, analysis, synthesis, and action. In the assessment phase, the respiratory care practitioner gathers information from patient charts and through interview, physical examination, and patient testing (such as PEFR). Analysis relates pathophysiology to patient data. To develop a successful treatment plan, the RCP must have a thorough understanding of normal physiology and how disease states alter this functioning. Assessment data and pathophysiology are then synthesized to develop a respiratory care plan through the use of therapist-driven protocols. Implementation of the plan is carried out in the action phase.

12. Pathophysiology deals with the dynamic aspects of a disease process. It is the study of the biological and physical manifestations of disease as they correlate with underlying abnormalities and physiologic disturbances.

13. Obstructive disorders are characterized by a blockage, or obstruction, to air flow. They are identified by a reduction in expiratory flowrates measured on pulmonary function studies. Conditions in this category include emphysema, chronic bronchitis, asthma, bronchiectasis, and cystic fibrosis. Restrictive disorders are characterized by increased stiffness of the lungs, thorax or both. They are identified by reduced lung volumes measured on pulmonary function studies. Conditions in this category include: extrapulmonary diseases such as amyotrophic lateral sclerosis (ALS), Guillain-Barré syndrome, myasthenia gravis, kyphosis and scoliosis; pleural disorders such as pleural effusion and pneumothorax; atelectasis; lung parenchymal infections; and pulmonary fibrosis.

14. An understanding of pathophysiology allows the RCP to make decisions about the patient's care plan based on the underlying disease or disorder rather than the symptoms alone. For example, treatment of dyspnea will differ depending on whether it is caused by airway obstruction or hypoxemia. For obstructive disease, an attempt would be made to reverse the obstruction; for hypoxemia, the treatment would be supplemental oxygen.

15. T
16. F
17. T
18. T
19. F
20. F
21. F
22. C
23. F
24. E
25. A
26. D
27. B

Posttest Answers

1. d
2. c
3. b
4. c
5. d
6. d
7. a
8. b
9. a
10. d

▬ Unit 1: Oxygen Therapy ▬▬▬▬▬▬▬▬▬▬▬▬▬

Topic 1: Oxygenation

1. mild hypoxemia: PaO_2 less than 80 mm Hg
   moderate hypoxemia: PaO_2 less than 60 mm Hg
   severe hypoxemia: PaO_2 less than 40 mm Hg

2. A PaO_2 of less than 40 mm Hg is considered a threat to tissue oxygenation because it results in a diminished driving force for oxygen in the systemic capillaries. A PaO_2 this low also increases hemoglobin's affinity for oxygen. These two factors combined result in less movement of oxygen molecules from systemic capillaries to the extracellular fluid compartment.

3. Uncorrected hypoxemia refers to a PaO_2 that remains less than 60 mm Hg despite increased inspired oxygen concentrations. Corrected hypoxemia is a PaO_2 of more than 60 mm Hg and less than 100 mm Hg on oxygen. Excessively corrected hypoxemia is a PaO_2 less than the minimal predicted normal at room air for that oxygen concentration but greater than 100 mm Hg. In other words, oxygen therapy is needed but can be decreased because the hypoxemia has been excessively corrected.

4. As a person ages the alveolar degenerative process continues, resulting in a decrease in the efficiency of the lungs to oxygenate the blood. This leads to decreased oxygen tensions in the arterial blood. A general guideline for determining the normal PaO_2 value for patients between 60 and 90 years of age is to subtract 1 mm Hg from the minimal PaO_2 of 80 mm Hg for every year over 60.

5. Cyanosis is the bluish coloration of the skin, mucous membranes, and nail beds. The presence of cyanosis correlates with at least 5 g/dL of reduced hemoglobin. Cyanosis is not considered to be a reliable indication of hypoxemia due to a number of factors. First, clinical detection varies among observers. Lighting conditions can affect the ability to detect conditions. Colors surrounding the patient such as blue sheets or blankets can affect patient coloration. Additionally, the absence of cyanosis does not necessarily indicate the absence of hypoxemia. Anemic patients can suffer hypoxemia with out showing signs of cyanosis while patients with polycythemia can manifest cyanosis with minimal hypoxemia and adequate tissue oxygenation.

6. Refractory hypoxemia is hypoxemia that does not respond significantly to oxygen therapy.

7. Oxygen is primarily transported in the blood bound to hemoglobin. It is also transported as a dissolved gas in the blood plasma in a smaller proportion.

8. The four physiologic causes of hypoxemia are hypoxemic hypoxia, anemic hypoxia, circulatory hypoxia, and histotoxic hypoxia. Hypoxemic hypoxia, also known as anoxic (hypoxic) hypoxemia,

refers to the condition in which the PaO_2 and CaO_2 are abnormally low. This type of hypoxemia results from three physiologic mechanisms: hypoventilation, $\dot{V}/\dot{Q}$ mismatch, and right-to-left shunt. Anemic hypoxia is a type of hypoxia in which the oxygen tension in the arterial blood is normal but the oxygen carrying capacity of the blood is inadequate. Anemic hypoxia can result from an absolute hemoglobin deficiency due to inadequate erythropoiesis, or loss of red blood cells (e.g., hemorrhage). Relative hemoglobin deficiencies are also responsible for anemic hypoxia. Examples of relative hemoglobin deficiencies would include carboxyhemoglobinemia and methemoglobinemia. Circulatory hypoxemia results when the arterial blood that reaches the tissues has the normal oxygen tension and content but the blood volume and, therefore, the amount of oxygen is inadequate to meet the needs of the tissues. This can occur with circulatory failure (shock) and local reduction in perfusion (ischemia). Histotoxic hypoxia is the condition in which the tissue cells are unable to utilize the oxygen delivered to them. Clinically, the PaO_2 and oxygen content are normal but the tissue cells themselves are extremely hypoxic. Cyanide poisoning is an example of histotoxic hypoxia.

9. The oxygen dissociation curve is shifted to the right with acidosis, hypercapnia, fever, and elevated concentrations of 2,3-DPG. It is shifted to the left with alkalosis, hypocapnia, decreased body temperature, decreased concentrations of 2,3-DPG, fetal hemoglobin, and carboxyhemoglobin.

10. Shifting the curve to the right decreases loading of oxygen in the lungs and facilitates unloading of oxygen at the tissues. When the curve is shifted to the left loading of oxygen in the lungs is facilitated and unloading of oxygen at the tissues is decreased.

11. PaO_2 of 30: SaO_2 60%
PaO_2 of 60: SaO_2 90%
PaO_2 of 90: SaO_2 97%

When looking at the oxygen dissociation curve and the three examples you should see that at high SaO_2s there is little change in SaO_2 with large changes in arterial PO_2. At low SaO_2s, small changes in PaO_2 can result in large changes in SaO_2.

12. Oxygen capacity is the maximum amount of oxygen that can combine with hemoglobin and dissolve in the plasma at a given PaO_2. Oxygen content reflects the actual amount of oxygen combined with hemoglobin and dissolved in the plasma.

13. Patient A = (1.34 x 16 x .95) + (90 x 0.003) = 20.64
Patient B = (1.34 x 8 x .95) + (90 x 0.003) = 10.45
Patient B has significantly less oxygen available for use by the tissues due to anemia.

14. Oxygen delivery to the tissues is dependent upon a number of factors including hemoglobin concentration, uptake of oxygen by the pulmonary blood, transport of oxygen in the arterial blood (including blood volume and tissue perfusion), diffusion of oxygen from the capillary bed into the tissues and diffusion from the tissues into the cells.

15. Deadspace-producing diseases and disorders include pulmonary embolus, decreased cardiac output, CNS abnormalities, emphysema, acute pulmonary hypertension, increased work of breathing, sedation, general anesthesia, positive pressure ventilation, and positive end-expiratory pressure.

16. Shunt-producing diseases and disorders include pulmonary edema, atelectasis, pulmonary tumors, pneumothorax, pneumonia, partial airway obstruction, pulmonary fibrosis, congenital heart disease, vascular lung disease, and intrapulmonary fistula.

17. Compensatory mechanisms seen in people with *chronic* hypoxemia include secondary polycythemia and pulmonary hypertension. Chronic hypoxemia stimulates the production of erythropoietin which stimulates the increased production of red blood cells. The increase of red blood cells results in an increased oxygen carrying capacity.

18. Compensatory mechanisms seen in people with *acute* hypoxemia include tachycardia, tachypnea, and increased blood pressure.

19. Clinical signs of hypoxemia include the hemodynamic compensatory mechanisms associated with stress, such as increased heart rate, increased respiratory rate, and increased blood pressure. In addition the patient may exhibit altered mental status, restlessness, and cyanosis.

20. The amount of oxygen delivered to the tissue beds is dependent on a number of factors, including the body's ability to oxygenate the blood; the type, function, and saturation of hemoglobin; the cardiac output; and local tissue perfusion.

21. As pulmonary disease progresses and arterial blood gases deteriorate, there comes a point when the $PaCO_2$ levels will have little effect on ventilatory drive. With chronically elevated $PaCO_2$ levels, the stimulus to breathe becomes lack of oxygen instead of increased carbon dioxide, which is the normal stimulus for respiration. The peripheral chemoreceptors are stimulated when the PaO_2 is below 60 mm Hg and the SaO_2 is about 80%. This situation is known as the hypoxic drive. These patients require carefully controlled FIO_2s (e.g., 24% or 28% air-entrainment mask) to prevent raising PaO_2 and SaO_2 high enough to depress the hypoxic drive.

22. Normal. Ventilation and perfusion are equally matched.
    Dead space. Ventilation without perfusion.
    Shunt. Perfusion without ventilation.
    Silent unit. No perfusion or ventilation.

23. T
24. T
25. T
26. F
27. T
28. F
29. T
30. F
31. T
32. T
33. T
34. T
35. T
36. F
37. F

Topic 2: Oxygen Delivery

38. The overall goal of oxygen therapy is to maintain adequate tissue oxygenation while lessening cardiac work and the work of breathing.

39. When respiratory care practitioners titrate oxygen they change the liter flow or oxygen concentration of the oxygen delivery device to maintain a predetermined minimal SpO_2 or PaO_2. This should be done according to hospital protocol. For example, when the protocol states "titrate the FIO_2 to maintain the SpO_2 to greater than or equal to 95%," the therapist would raise or lower the FIO_2 delivered to meet the stated goal.

40. A variable-performance device delivers oxygen to the patient but does not provide all the patient's inspired gas needs. Variable-performance devices are also known as low flow oxygen systems. A fixed-performance device provides a constant FIO_2 by meeting or exceeding the patient's inspiratory flow demand. The fixed-performance devices are also known as high flow systems.

41. A. Nasal catheter, variable-performance device
    B. Air-entrainment mask (Venti-mask), fixed-performance device
    C. Nasal cannula, variable-performance device
    D. Simple mask, variable-performance device
    E. Non-rebreathing mask, variable-performance device (fixed-performance only when leak-free)

42. Advantages of a nasal cannula include the following: it is simple to put in place; it allows for speech and eating; it does not make the patient feel claustrophobic; it causes little or no discomfort; and it is relatively unobtrusive. Disadvantages of the nasal cannula include: FIO_2 variations with rate, depth and pattern of breathing; tendency of high flowrates to dry and irritate nasal mucosa; pressure ulcers on the nose, ears, and face; and limitation of the FIO_2 to low and moderate levels.

43. The air-to-oxygen ratio for a 35% air-entrainment device is 5:1. The total ratio parts is 6; at 10 L/min the total flow would be (6 x 10 L/min) 60 L/min. During normal quiet breathing the flowrate needed to meet inspiratory demand seldom exceeds 30 L/min. The peak inspiratory flow can easily double or triple in acutely ill patients. As a general rule of thumb, it is suggested the total output flow of oxygen devices be at least 60 L/min to provide the total flow required by the patient and to ensure that the device provides accurate FIO_2s. In this case the total output of the 35% air-entrainment mask is sufficient.

44. Air-entrainment masks are fixed-performance devices that provide the patient with a stable FIO_2. COPD patients who may hypoventilate when exposed to high FIO_2s should not use variable-performance devices during acute exacerbations of their condition or while their breathing pattern is irregular. The air-entrainment mask will provide a stable FIO_2 despite their changing ventilatory pattern or requirements.

45. Disadvantages of oxygen masks include the following: increased risk of aspiration if the patient vomits; discomfort (tight fit, warm); more difficulties in eating, drinking, and communication; and feelings of claustrophobia. Oxygen masks are often tolerated less well than the nasal cannula.

46. The mask is placed on the patient's face and adjusted to provide a good facial seal. The flowrate required is generally between 6 and 10 L/min and depends on the patient's inspiratory flow. The reservoir bag should remain full and should never fully deflate during patient inspiration.

47. Advantages of reservoir masks include the following: moderate to high oxygen concentrations are delivered and the masks are inexpensive, disposable, and easily applied. The disadvantages include the fact that these variable-performance devices are relatively uncomfortable and they lack the good seal necessary to permit room-air dilution.

48. The harmful effects of oxygen therapy include oxygen toxicity, oxygen-induced hypoventilation, retinopathy of prematurity, absorption atelectasis, depression of ciliary activity and/or leukocyte function, and altered surfactant production/activity.

49. Factors that hasten onset or increase the severity of oxygen toxicity include increased age, steroid administration, catecholamines, protein malnutrition, Vitamin C, E or A deficiency, trace element deficiency, elevated serum iron, bleomycin or Adriamycin, paraquat herbicide exposure, and hyperthermia.

50. The clinical picture of patient exposed to high oxygen concentrations is similar to that seen in diffuse bronchopneumonia. Patients complain of substernal chest pain and tightness. Vital capacity and lung compliance decrease. Chest radiograph reveals patchy infiltrates and there are areas of low V/Q ratios and physiologic shunting. In the late stages hyaline membranes form in the alveolar regions, followed by development of pulmonary fibrosis and pulmonary hypertension.

51. Most studies find that oxygen concentrations up to 50% are safe. However, contrary reports exist. It is therefore best to use the lowest amount possible to treat hypoxemia.

52. According to the AARC Clinical Practice Guideline for oxygen therapy in the home or extended care facility, oxygen therapy is indicated for home use when there is documented hypoxemia in adults, children and infants older than 28 days as evidenced by (1) PaO_2 less than or equal to 55 mm Hg or SaO_2 less than or equal to 88% in subjects breathing room air or (2) PaO_2 of 56 to 59 mm Hg or SaO_2 or SpO_2 of less than or equal to 89% in association with specific clinical conditions (cor pulmonale, congestive heart failure, or erythrocythemia with hematocrit greater than 56).

53. T
54. T
55. T
56. F
57. T
58. F
59. T
60. F
61. T
62. T
63. F
64. T
65. F
66. T
67. F
68. D
69. B
70. A
71. F
72. H

Topic 3: Analysis of Oxygenation

73. Pulse oximetry incorporates two physical principles of operation—spectrophotometry and photo-plethysmography—to determine the level of oxygen saturation in the blood. Using two wavelengths of light, red and infrared, the degree of change in light absorption is used to determine the relative proportions of oxyhemoglobin and deoxyhemoglobin. Plethysmographic technology is used to differentiate between venous and arterial blood for analysis.

74. The limitations affecting the accuracy of pulse oximeters include the following: skin pigmentation, vascular dyes, motion artifact, abnormal hemoglobin (e.g., carboxyhemoglobin), low perfusion states, anemia, light dilution, nail polish/coverings (with finger probe), inability to quantitate the degree of hyperoxemia present, calibration, and accuracy.

75. Carboxyhemoglobin results in an overestimation of actual saturation because the pulse oximeter cannot distinguish carboxyhemoglobin from oxyhemoglobin.

76. Indications for pulse oximetry measurement include the following: the need to monitor the adequacy of arterial oxyhemoglobin saturation, the need to quantitate the response of arterial oxyhemoglobin saturation to therapeutic intervention or to a diagnostic procedure, and the need to comply with mandated regulations or recommendations by authoritative groups.

77. Relative contraindications to pulse oximetry include the presence of a need for measurement of pH, $PaCO_2$, total hemoglobin, abnormal hemoglobins, and presence of the factors noted in answer 74 above.

78. A pulse oximetry reading can be validated by comparing the reading to that of the co-oximeter. In addition, when comparison to the co-oximeter is not feasible the pulse recorded on the pulse oximeter should be compared to the patient's actual pulse rate.

79. SpO_2 documentation should include date, time of reading, pulse oximeter reading, patient's position and/or activity level, inspired oxygen concentration/oxygen flowrate and oxygen device in use, results of simultaneously drawn ABG, clinical appearance of the patient (e.g., cyanosis), skin temperature, agreement between pulse rate by oximeter and actual rate, and any other information that would detail the conditions under which the pulse oximeter readings were obtained.

80. F
81. T
82. T
83. T
84. F

Topic 4: Follow-up to Mr. Feder

85. According to the AARC Clinical Practice Guideline for oxygen therapy in the acute care hospital, patients should be monitored when placed on oxygen therapy as follows: perform a clinical assessment including, but not limited to, cardiac, pulmonary, and neurologic status; assess physiologic parameters; measure oxygen tensions or saturations in any patient treated with oxygen. This should be done within 12 hours of initiation with FIO_2 less than 0.40, within 8 hours with FIO_2s greater than or equal to 0.40 (including postanesthesia recovery), within 72 hours in acute myocardial infarction, within 2 hours for any patient with the principal diagnosis of COPD, and within 1 hour for the neonate. In Mr. Feder's case, he should be assessed within 2 hours because of the diagnosis of COPD.

86. After 24 hours of oxygen therapy an assessment of Mr. Feder, including but not limited to cardiac, pulmonary, and neurologic status is warranted. This would include assessment of vital signs, mental status, and SpO_2. When following the protocol on page 245, the oxygen can be titrated by decreasing the oxygen by 1 L/min to room air as long as the oxygen is not needed for exercise and the SpO_2 is greater than or equal to 92%. If oxygen therapy is stopped the patient should be checked the following shift. Oxygen can be discontinued at this time as long as the SpO_2 remains greater than or equal to 92%. Practitioners should follow the protocols at their institutions when evaluating and changing oxygen therapy.

87. In this scenario, Mr. Feder seems to be improving, and a trial of decreasing the oxygen therapy is indicated. Hospital protocols should be followed and the patient's SpO_2 monitored.

88. When the SpO_2 cannot be maintained at the prescribed level, the physician must be notified immediately. Arterial blood gas analysis and alternate forms of therapy (e.g., CPAP) may be needed to treat the refractory hypoxemia.

89. Cardiac patients are maintained at a higher SpO_2 of 95% or within physician-specified limits. The higher value in this case is a safeguard against the limited cardiac reserve this patient group often has.

90. Need for home oxygen therapy is determined by the presence of clinical indicators such as documented hypoxemia as evidenced by (1) PaO_2 less than or equal to 55 mm Hg or SaO_2 less than or equal to 88% in subjects breathing room air or (2) PaO_2 of 56-59 mm Hg or SaO_2 or SpO_2 of less than or equal to 89% in association with specific clinical conditions (e.g., cor pulmonale, congestive heart failure, or polycythemia with hematocrit greater than 56). In Mr. Feder's case, this would mean a PaO_2 less than or equal to 55 mm Hg or SaO_2 less than or equal to 88% breathing room air. Concurrent pulse oximetry values must be documented and reconciled with the results of the baseline blood gas analysis if future assessment is to involve pulse oximetry.

91. In this situation the patient has vital signs denoting significant stress. His respiratory rate is greater than 25 and his SpO_2 is less than 88%. Following the protocol on page 245, this patient should be placed on a high-flow system ensuring his inspiratory demands are met. The oxygen concentration should be titrated to maintain a SpO_2 greater than or equal to 92% or within physician specified limits. The patient should be reassessed within 8 hours.

Posttest Answers

1. b
2. c
3. a
4. b
5. c
6. c
7. a
8. d
9. a
10. b
11. d
12. d
13. b
14. a
15. a
16. b
17. b
18. a
19. d
20. b
21. a
22. b
23. c
24. a
25. d

Unit 2: Aerosol Therapy

Topic 1: Aerosol Therapy Equipment

1. An aerosol is liquid or solid particles of a substance suspended in a gas.

2. The six factors that affect the deposition of aerosol particles are gravity, kinetic activity, particle inertia, physical nature of particles, temperature and humidity, and ventilatory patterns.

3. The MMAD is the mean mass aerodynamic diameter, defined as the distribution of particle diameter around which the mass of particles is equally distributed with 50% of the particles heavier and 50% lighter.

4. Aerosol particles with an MMAD of less than or equal to 5 microns tend to deposit in the lungs while aerosol particles greater than 5 microns impact on the upper airway.

5. An MDI is a pressurized cartridge and mouthpiece assembly used for self-administration of exact dosages of aerosolized medications.

6. The float test can be done to estimate the remaining amount of medication in an MDI canister. The canister is floated in a container of water. A full canister will sink to the bottom. As the canister

empties it will start to float to the top. Empty canisters float on their side horizontally along the top of the container of water.

7. DPIs are small, portable, and practical. In addition, they do not use chlorofluorocarbons. Because they are breath actuated, they minimize hand-breath coordination problems.

8. Disadvantages of DPIs include the following: (1) the limited number of drugs available in this form, (2) patients must be able to generate a sufficient inspiratory flowrate to actuate the device, and (3) powder medications can be affected by humidity.

9. One technique used to minimize drug loss with small volume nebulizers is intermittent nebulization using a patient-controlled finger port to direct gas to the nebulizer only during inspiration. A second technique is to add approximately six inch (50 ml) length of aerosol tubing as an expiratory reservoir to the nebulizer.

10. A study by Hughes and Saez in 1987 found that the optimal placement of the nebulizer is in the inspiratory limb at the manifold of the ventilator circuit, about 18 inches from the patient wye.

11. Large volume nebulizers are very useful when traditional dosing is ineffective. Large volume nebulizers can provide continuous therapy, even while the patient sleeps.

12. One problem associated with continuous nebulization of medication using large volume nebulizers is that the concentration of drug increases over time as evaporation occurs. Patients should be monitored closely for signs of drug toxicity during continuous nebulization therapy.

13. According to the AARC Clinical Practice Guideline for selection of aerosol delivery device, one indication for aerosol therapy is the need to deliver medications from the following classes to the lungs: beta adrenergic agents, anticholinergic agents (antimuscarinics), anti-inflammatory agents (e.g., corticosteroids), mediator-modifying compounds (e.g., cromolyn sodium), mucokinetics, and antibiotics. In addition, indications for aerosol therapy can include enhancement of secretion clearance, sputum induction, humidification of inspired gases, and the treatment of upper airway inflammation with unheated bland aerosols.

14. Hazards/complications of aerosol delivery include: malfunction of the device and/or improper technique which may result in underdosing or overdosing; side effects of specific pharmacologic agents; cardiotoxic effects of Freon; an idiosyncratic response that may be a problem with excessive use of MDI; and Freon's potential effect on the ozone layer of the atmosphere. Repeated exposure to aerosols has been reported to produce asthmatic symptoms in some caregivers.

15. Limitations of MDI therapy include environmental concerns of chlorofluorocarbons such as Freon; incorrect technique; and inadequate instruction. In addition, when spacers are used, the cost increases, and the device is more bulky than the MDI alone.

16. Limitations of DPI dosing include: patients must load each dose for most medications; reduced inspiratory flow (less than 60 L/min) can lead to reduced deposition; powder can irritate the airway; and humidity may cause clumping of powder particles.

17. Limitations of small volume nebulizers include: administration by this method is labor- and time-intensive; they are less portable; they require a compressed-gas source or electricity; they are vulnerable to contamination; and lack of convenience may affect patient compliance.

18. Limitations of ultrasonic nebulizer therapy include: the cost of the device, mechanical reliability, the need for an electric power source, and susceptibility to contamination.

19. MDI with an accessory device should be the first method considered for administration of aerosol to the airway because of its proven therapeutic efficacy, variety of available medications, and cost-effectiveness.

20. Monitoring of aerosol therapy should include performance of the device, technique of device application, and assessment of patient response, including changes in vital signs and lung function measurements.

21. Infection control procedures for aerosol delivery include the following universal precautions: (1) small volume and large volume nebulizers are for single patient use or subjected to high-level disinfection between patients, (2) these devices should be changed or subjected to high-level disinfection at approximately 24-hour intervals, (3) medications should be handled aseptically, (4) tap water should never be used as a diluent, (5) medications from multidose sources must be handled aseptically and the multidose bottle should be discarded after 24 hours (unless specified otherwise by the manufacturer), and (6) MDI accessory devices are for single patient use only and cleaning is based on aesthetic criteria. There are no documented concerns with contamination of medication in MDI canisters.

22. Criteria for choosing a small-volume aerosol delivery device over the other devices include the following: inability of the patient to follow instructions or perform a breath-hold, poor inspiratory capacity, tachypnea or unstable respiratory pattern, and the need to aerosolize drugs not in MDI or DPI form.

23. The ultrasonic nebulizer uses standard electric current to produce sound waves that are used to create the aerosol. The ultrasonic nebulizer incorporates the use of a piezoelectric transducer which changes shape when an electric charge is applied. The electric current causes vibrations at the same frequency as the electric charge. This determines the particle size of the aerosol as the liquid is broken up at its surface. The amplitude determines the number of particles produced (aerosol output).

24. The small-particle aerosol generator (SPAG) is a device manufactured by ICN Pharmaceuticals specifically for the administration of Virazole (ribavirin). This device is unique because it incorporates a drying chamber with its own flow control to produce a stable aerosol. The drying chamber creates an almost monodisperse output with aerosol particles mostly between 1.2 and 1.4 microns.

25. The Babbington nebulizer uses a high-pressure gas source directed inside a glass sphere with a small opening from which the gas can exit. The outside of the sphere is covered with a thin film of liquid to be aerosolized. As the gas leaves the sphere it ruptures the film of liquid creating aerosol particles. A baffle is incorporated to assist in creating the appropriate particle size and uniformity.

26. T
27. T
28. F
29. T
30. T
31. T
32. T
33. T
34. T
35. T
36. F
37. T
38. F
39. F
40. T
41. d
42. c
43. e
44. g
45. f
46. a
47. b

Topic 2: Bland Aerosol Administration

48. Bland aerosol therapy includes the delivery of sterile water or hypotonic, isotonic, or hypertonic saline in aerosol form.

49. The indications for bland aerosol administration include the presence of upper airway edema; laryngotracheobronchitis; subglottic edema; postextubation edema; postoperative management of the upper airway; the presence of a bypassed upper airway; and the need for sputum induction.

50. Contraindications to bland aerosol administration include bronchoconstriction and history of airway hyperresponsiveness.

51. The hazards and complications of bland aerosol administration include the following: wheezing or bronchospasm; bronchoconstriction when used with an artificial airway; infection; overhydration; patient discomfort; and caregiver exposure to droplet nuclei of *Mycobacterium tuberculosis* or other airborne contagion produced as a consequence of patient coughing, particularly during sputum induction.

52. Patient monitoring is tailored to patient needs. It may include assessment of the patient's subjective report of discomfort, such as dyspnea or restlessness; heart rate and rhythm; blood pressure; respiratory rate, pattern, and mechanics; accessory muscle use; sputum production amount, color, consistency, and odor; skin color; breath sounds; and pulse oximetry.

53. T
54. F
55. T
56. T
57. T
58. T
59. T
60. F
61. T
62. T

Topic 3: Follow-up to Mr. Carr

63. When determining how an aerosolized medication is to be delivered to a patient, the respiratory care practitioner must first determine the need for therapy. Assuming the medication is in fact indicated, the form of the medication may limit the choice of delivery. Next the efficiency of the spontaneous breath should be determined. If patients do not have a sufficient inspiratory volume due to tachypnea, small volume nebulizer might be the method of choice. If the volume is decreased due to weakness then IPPB might be a better choice for delivery. Breath hold may also be evaluated in an effort to determine the delivery method. A 6-second or greater hold indicates the patient may be able to use an MDI. Patients with a poor breath hold may be better served with small volume nebulizer therapy. Patients not responsive to scheduled treatments may be candidates for continuous nebulization via large volume nebulizers.

64. Since Mr. Carr exhibited significant tachypnea in this scenario, the protocol advises that the patient receive the drug by small volume nebulization as opposed to MDI.

65. Now that Mr. Carr's respiratory rate is within the normal range and he is calmer, he is more likely able to perform an adequate breath hold and could be evaluated for MDI therapy. Education on proper technique and follow-up would be needed.

66. Even with a spacer device, the patient must coordinate actuation of the MDI with inhalation. Exhalation immediately after the MDI is actuated can clear the aerosol from the device, wasting the dose to the atmosphere.

67. In this scenario Mr. Carr's pre-treatment peak flow was 350 L/min and his post-treatment peak flow was 460 L/min. The percent change is calculated:

$$\frac{460 - 350}{350} \times 100 = 31\%$$

This is a significant improvement and the therapy should be continued.

68. Mr. Carr is responsive to the medications he has received. It may be time to deliver the medication using MDI. His technique should be evaluated and monitored closely. Mr. Carr would also benefit from a comprehensive asthma education program.

69. When instructing a patient on the optimal technique for use of an MDI without an accessory device, the respiratory care practitioner should include the following information: warm the MDI to hand or body temperature; assemble the device making sure there are no objects that could block the out flow; shake the canister vigorously; hold canister upright, placing it two fingers away from an open mouth*; after a normal exhalation, begin to inspire slowly while actuating the MDI, continue to inhale a full deep breath, hold the breath for a count of ten, wait one minute (or as directed by your physician) between actuations.
   * Some protocols have the patient place the MDI in the mouth with the lips closed around the mouthpiece as opposed to the open-mouth technique. In this case, hospital protocol should be followed.

Posttest Answers

1. b
2. c
3. d
4. a
5. c
6. c
7. b
8. c
9. a
10. d
11. b
12. d
13. a
14. d
15. b
16. c
17. d
18. a
19. a
20. c
21. b
22. a
23. d
24. b
25. a

▬ **Unit 3: Secretion Management** ▬▬▬▬▬▬▬▬▬▬

Topic 1: Mucociliary Transport

1. Normal respiratory mucus clearance is accomplished by the mucociliary escalator. The mucociliary escalator has two basic components known as the cilia and the mucus blanket. The ciliated cells of the mucosal lining are essential in clearing and defending the respiratory tract. The cilia beat in a rhythmic manner called the metachronal wave. This action propels surface debris from the bronchioles up to the larynx in the direction toward the pharynx. The success of ciliary action is dependent on the mucus layer. The mucus layer has two components called the gel and sol layers. The sol layer lies on the mucosal surface and contains high concentrations of water. The effectiveness of the cilia to move debris depends on the ability of the cilia to beat and mobilize the sol layer. The function of the gel layer is to adhere to debris.

2. a. respiratory cilia
   b. gel layer
   c. sol layer

3. Some of the factors that disrupt normal respiratory mucus clearance include dehydration, infection, placement of artificial airways, suctioning, immobile cilia syndrome, inhaled anesthesia, increased FIO_2, and cigarette smoking.

4. A normal cough has four distinct phases. A cough begins either voluntarily or with the irritation phase. An irritation provokes sensory fibers to send afferent impulses to the cough center. The stimulus can be many different irritants such as a foreign body, an infection, inhaled chemicals or cold air. Once the afferent impulses are processed in the cough center, a deep inspiration is initiated. Following the deep inspiration, efferent impulses cause glottic closure and a forceful contraction of the expiratory muscles. This results in a rapid increase in pleural and alveolar pressures. This third phase is called the compression phase. The final phase is the expulsion phase. During the expulsion phase the glottis opens and a large pressure gradient is established between the alveoli and the airway opening. The pressure gradient, along with continued contraction of the expiratory muscles, results in an expulsive flow of gas from the lungs.

5. a. irritation
   b. inspiration
   c. compression
   d. expulsion

6. The segments of the lungs include the following:
   right upper lobe: apical, posterior, and anterior.
   right middle lobe: lateral and medial.
   right lower lobe: superior, medial basal, anterior basal, lateral basal, and posterior basal.
   left upper lobe: apical posterior, anterior, superior, and inferior. The superior and inferior segments are known as the lingula.
   left lower lobe: superior, anterior basal, lateral basal, posterior basal.

7. T
8. T
9. T
10. F
11. T

Topic 2: Pneumonia

12. *Streptococcus pneumoniae, Hemophilus influenzae, chlamydia* species, *Mycoplasma pneumoniae*, or common viruses account for 95% of the pneumonias developed in adults in the usual community setting.

13. Alveolar, also known as acinar, has radiographic features described as fluffy shadows that result from fluid accumulation in the distal airspaces of the lung. Interstitial, also known as reticular, has radiographic features described as shadows that form a lacey network of linear markings. These markings may reflect increased inflammatory material or chronic changes such as fibrosis. Bronchopneumonia has radiographic features described as scattered fluffy shadows that tend to be patchy and follow the distribution of the central conducting airways. Lobar pneumonia has radiographic features that are described as confluent shadows that usually end at pleural surfaces and usually involve entire lobes or segments. Air bronchograms are often seen. Necrotizing pneumonia has radiographic features described as lucencies depicting pneumonia in which cavities are seen.

14. *Streptococcus pneumoniae*, also called *pneumococcus*, is the cause of most bacterial pneumonias in the normal host, the elderly and in patients with chronic diseases. The onset is most often sudden, with patients complaining of high fever, shaking chills, pleuritic chest pain, and a productive cough. The sputum is mucopurulent or "rusty" blood streaked. Dyspnea and tachypnea are also common. Physical examination reveals decreased chest excursion, crackles and possible friction rub on the involved side. Gram's stain of the sputum reveals gram-positive organisms that on culture will be *pneumococci*. The patient's white blood cell count is usually elevated. The chest radiograph may be unremarkable, except for haziness in the involved area of the lung. Consolidation, if it develops, may be a lobar pattern. Treatment of *pneumococcal* pneumonia consists of selection of an appropriate antibiotic (e.g., penicillin G or erythromycin), bed rest, hydration, chest physical therapy, and oxygen therapy as needed.

15. Although there are over two hundred different viruses known to cause respiratory tract infections, the following are the best known: influenza, respiratory syncytial virus (RSV), adenoviruses, *cytomegalovirus* (CMV).

16. Examples of conditions in which host defenses are impaired include the following: AIDS, alcoholism, altered mental status, antacid therapy, antibiotic therapy, ARDS, COPD, cytotoxic chemotherapy, diabetes, histamine blocker therapy, immunosuppressive therapy, increasing age, leukemia, malignancy, mechanical ventilation, renal failure, thoracoabdominal surgery, tracheal intubation, and viral infections.

17. A patient with lobar pneumonia and pulmonary consolidation would demonstrate dullness to percussion, increased tactile fremitus, egophony, bronchophony, whispered pectoriloquy, bronchial breath sounds, and crackles.

18. Unusual organisms known to cause pneumonia in the normal host include the following: *Legionella, Mycobacterium*, group A *streptococcus, meningococcus*, and *B. anthracis*. In the abnormal host, *enterococcus*, group B *streptococcus, Aspergillus, Nocardia, P. carinii, cytomegalovirus*, and *Mycobacteria* are known causes of pneumonia.

19. Organisms commonly causing nosocomial pneumonia include gram-positive cocci, fungi, viruses, *Pneumocystis, Legionella* species, and other gram-negative bacilli.

20. Colonization is the process by which microorganisms establish a presence and grow, but it does not necessarily indicate a pathological response. Infection is the invasion of the body by pathogenic microorganisms causing disease by local cellular injury, secretion of a toxin, or antigen-antibody reaction in the host.

21. b
22. j
23. i
24. c
25. d
26. g
27. f
28. h
29. T
30. F
31. T
32. T
33. T
34. F
35. T
36. T
37. T
38. T

Topic 3: Chest Physical Therapy

39. Goals of chest physical therapy include the following: prevent the accumulation of secretions; improve mobilization and drainage of secretions; promote relaxation to improve breathing patterns; promote improved respiratory function; developing respiratory strength and endurance; improve cardiopulmonary exercise tolerance; teach bronchial hygiene programs to patients with chronic respiratory dysfunction in airway clearance.

40. The term chest physical therapy has traditionally referred to postural drainage, percussion, and vibration. More recently what is considered to be chest physical therapy techniques has expanded to include many additional procedures, such as directed cough, segmental breathing, autogenic drainage, and PEP therapy.

41. The indications for turning include the inability or reluctance to change body position. Mechanical ventilation, drug induced paralysis, and neuromuscular disease are all examples of factors which limit a patients' mobility and put them at risk for secretion retention. These patients would benefit from frequent changes in body position.

42. The indications for postural drainage include the following: evidence or suggestion of difficulty with secretion clearance; presence of atelectasis caused by (or suspected of being caused by) mucus plugging; diagnosis of diseases such as cystic fibrosis, bronchiectasis, or cavitating lung disease.

43. The indications for external manipulation of the thorax include sputum volume or consistency suggesting a need for additional manipulation to assist movement of secretions in patients receiving postural drainage. External manipulation refers to techniques such as percussion and vibration.

44. There are a number of acute conditions for which scientific evidence supports chest physical therapy techniques as treatment. These include acutely ill patients with copious amounts of secretions, patients with acute respiratory failure and clinical signs of retained secretions, patients with acute lobar atelectasis, and patients with $\dot{V}/\dot{Q}$ abnormalities due to infiltrate or consolidation.

45. The first of the two chronic conditions benefiting from chest physical therapy would include any condition resulting in chronic production of large volumes of sputum (greater than 25 to 30 ml of sputum per day). Patients with cystic fibrosis, bronchiectasis, and certain patients with chronic bronchitis would be included in this group. The second condition indicating the need for chest physical therapy includes COPD accompanied by inefficient breathing patterns and/or decreased exercise tolerance.

46. Evidence is mixed with regard to the use of chest physical therapy as preventative method of respiratory care. It has been suggested that preventative chest physical therapy may benefit patients at high risk for developing postoperative respiratory complications, patients with neuromuscular disorders that compromise the normal clearance of the respiratory tract, and chronic obstructive lung disease patients prone to exacerbations of their disease. Chest physical therapy has been used as a prophylactic mode of respiratory care for a variety of patient conditions. These include the prevention of postoperative complications in high risk populations, prevention of respiratory problems in patients with neuromuscular dysfunction increasing the risk of secretion retention, and for the prevention of exacerbations of chronic lung disease (e.g., cystic fibrosis).

47. The primary objectives of therapeutic positioning (turning) include the following: turning the patient who is unable or reluctant to do so, improving oxygenation related to positioning, and reducing atelectasis.

48. When respiratory care practitioners perform the initial assessment of a patient for chest physical therapy they might consider the following: analysis of the patient's chart, including the history of pulmonary problems causing increased secretions; chest assessment (inspection, auscultation, percussion and palpation); oxygenation status; chest radiograph indicating infiltrates or atelectasis; pulmonary function test results; effectiveness of the cough; sputum production; breathing pattern; vital signs; identification of respiratory therapy appliances that could enhance chest physical therapy; assessment of the degree of stress and tension exhibited by the patient; muscle strength training; joint range-of-motion testing.

49. The AARC Clinical Practice Guidelines include two absolute contraindications to postural drainage positioning. The absolute contraindications are head and neck injury until stabilized and active hemorrhage with hemodynamic instability.

50. Relative contraindications to postural drainage include the following: intracranial pressure greater than 20 mm Hg; recent spinal surgery or acute spinal injury; active hemoptysis; empyema; bronchopleural fistula; pulmonary edema associated with congestive heart failure; large pleural effusions; pulmonary embolism; aged/confused or anxious patients who do not tolerate position changes; rib fracture, with or without flail; surgical wound healing; uncontrolled hypertension; distended abdomen; esophageal surgery; uncontrolled airway at risk for aspiration.

51. When performing postural drainage, the patient's vital signs (including pulse, respiratory rate, and blood pressure) should be monitored. Oxygen saturation and electrocardiogram monitoring should also be monitored whenever this information is available. Chest auscultation should be performed before and after the therapy.

52. Outcome criteria that indicate a positive response to postural drainage include increase in sputum production, improvement in breath sounds, restoration of normal vital signs, resolution of abnormal chest radiograph, normalization in ABG values or oxygen saturation, improvement in mechanical ventilator variables (improved compliance/decreased resistance), and positive subjective responses by the patient concerning postural drainage.

53. When documenting a chest physical therapy session, the respiratory care practitioner should include the following: date, time of therapy, specific positions used, any modifications from standard procedure, patient tolerance, subjective and objective indicators of treatment effectiveness, oxygen therapy required, vital signs, monitoring done during therapy, patient education and the patient's therapeutic plan.

54. Segmental breathing is a technique designed to promote improved localized ventilation in a target area. Respiratory care practitioners would place their own or the patient's hand over the segment to be expanded. The patient is instructed to take a deep breath and push the hand away on inspiration. Slight pressure is applied during the exercise to provide reinforcement and encouragement of a full inspiration.

55. The lateral (unilateral or bilateral) breathing exercise is done to promote lateral costal expansion of the lower chest. The goal is to improve ventilation. Hands are placed on the side of the chest to be emphasized.

56. Pursed lip breathing is a technique that can be used to prolong one's expiratory phase. When the lips are pursed together and the patient breaths slowly through them, a positive back-pressure on the airways is created. This allows the patient to exhale with less early airway closure, allowing more volume to be exhaled. Encouraging patients to use the pursed lip breathing technique when they are dyspneic helps them regain control of their breathing.

57. Directed cough is a technique taught to patients and supervised to mimic the features of a successful spontaneous cough. This technique is successful in clearing secretions form the central airways.

58. The indications for directed cough are as follows: the need to clear retained secretions from central airways; the presence of atelectasis; to help prevent postoperative pulmonary complications; as a routine part of bronchial hygiene in patients with cystic fibrosis, bronchiectasis, chronic bronchitis, necrotizing pulmonary infection, or spinal cord injury; as a component of other bronchial hygiene therapies; to obtain sputum specimens for diagnostic analysis.

59. Postsurgical patients will benefit from coordinating the directed cough sessions with their prescribed pain medication. The patients will also benefit in "splinting" the operative site during the session.

60. The forced expiration technique consists of forced expirations from mid- to low-lung volume without closure of the glottis, followed by a period of diaphragmatic breathing and relaxation. This technique is a modification of the directed cough and its goal is to improve secretion clearance.

61. Positive expiratory pressure (PEP) therapy is a technique that incorporates expiratory resistance to help mobilize secretions. Patients exhale against resistance and, depending on their expiratory flow, create expiratory pressure. Studies have documented this technique to be effective in mobilizing secretions in patients with cystic fibrosis.

62. To minimize risk of desaturation, the respiratory care practitioner can monitor patients' oxygen saturations and vital signs and provide supplemental oxygen or increase the delivered FIO_2 as needed during chest physical therapy sessions.

63. According to the AARC Clinical Practice Guidelines, when a patient vomits during chest postural drainage, the therapy should be stopped. Clear the airway and suction as needed to maintain the airway. Oxygen can be administered. The patient should be returned to his or her previous resting position.

64. Changes in breath sounds from diminished pretreatment to adventitious sounds during or following therapy can be considered an improvement. The secretions may have moved into large airways and may be at the point in which they can be cleared with a good cough. The patient should be encouraged to clear the secretions, assisted in secretion removal as needed, and reevaluated.

65. Autogenic drainage is a technique used to facilitate secretion removal and is a modification of the directed cough. Autogenic drainage combines the technique of breathing at low lung volumes with an inspiratory hold and controlled exhalation. The goal is to obtain maximal expiratory airflow without causing airway collapse enhancing secretion removal.

66. The high-frequency chest wall compression system incorporates a variable air-pulse generator and an inflatable vest to promote secretion clearance.

67. Relaxation positioning offers patients a simple technique that facilitates the descent of the diaphragm by relaxing the abdominal muscles due to the forward position. In addition, by fixing the upper arms, the accessory muscles of inspiration work more efficiently. When patients focus their attention on the positioning and slow their breathing rate, they often experience a lessening in their sensation of shortness of breath. They will also have a decreased oxygen demand due to a decrease in work of breathing.

68. Diaphragmatic breathing is a technique used to promote greater use of the diaphragm and lessen the use of the accessory muscles. It is also called abdominal breathing.

69. e
70. d
71. c
72. b
73. a
74. T
75. T
76. T
77. T
78. T
79. F
80. F
81. F
82. T
83. F
84. T
85. T
86. F
87. T

Topic 4: Follow-up to Mr. Gonsalves

88. To evaluate the chest physical therapy performed on Mr. Gonsalves, the therapist should consider his sputum volume and character, chest radiograph, vital signs (including temperature), and ABG or oxygen saturation results.

89. Based on the fact the patient is no longer producing a large volume of sputum and the pneumonia is resolving, the chest postural drainage and percussion should be discontinued. The MDI and patient education (disease/pharmacology/smoking cessation) should be continued.

90. In this case the evaluation of outcome criteria supports continuing the chest physical therapy. The therapy has increased the patient's sputum production, resulting in a total daily amount of greater than 30 ml. The patient's subjective response is positive and his vital signs have normalized. With continued respiratory care, the chest radiograph and breath sounds should improve.

91. Dehydration must be considered when a respiratory care practitioner is making a determination on the effectiveness of chest physical therapy. Adequate systemic and airway hydration is necessary for effective mucociliary clearance. It may take 24 hours after a patient has been adequately hydrated before any evidence of increased sputum production is seen.

92. Considering the AARC Clinical Practice Guidelines, when dysrhythmia is noted on the ECG monitor, the correct intervention is to stop therapy, return the patient to previous resting position, and administer or increase oxygen delivered while contacting the physician.

Posttest Answers

1. c
2. b
3. a
4. b
5. c
6. d
7. a

8. c
9. d
10. a
11. b
12. c
13. d
14. c
15. a
16. d
17. b
18. c
19. d
20. c
21. c
22. b
23. d
24. d
25. a

Unit 4: Volume Expansion

Topic 1: Pathophysiology of Atelectasis

1. Airway obstruction and altered sigh mechanism are considered to be the two fundamental causes of atelectasis. Airway obstruction can be caused by mucosal edema, bronchospasm, foreign body, and retained secretions. Alveolar gas can become trapped in the alveoli distal to the obstruction. Over time the trapped gasses will enter the pulmonary circulation and alveolar collapse will occur. An abnormal sigh mechanism can result in a breathing pattern that produces few or no sigh breaths. Sigh breaths are needed to inflate alveoli beyond tidal breathing. These periodic deep breaths are believed to help the type II pneumocytes secrete surfactant. Surfactant is crucial in maintaining normal surface tension forces within the alveoli, preventing collapse. Abnormal sigh mechanisms have therefore been associated with the development of atelectasis.

2. There are many risk factors and clinical conditions that have been shown to contribute to the development of atelectasis. These may include smoking, increased age, dehydration, obesity, general debilitation or malnutrition, underlying pulmonary or cardiovascular disease, general anesthesia, thoracic surgery, upper abdominal surgery, postoperative pain, immobility, sedatives, muscle relaxants, and narcotic use.

3. Clinical signs of atelectasis include decreased chest expansion, dull percussion note, diminished breath sounds, and tactile fremitus.

4. The physiologic manifestations of atelectasis include reduced lung compliance, increased work of breathing, decreased functional residual capacity, increased pulmonary shunting, decreased arterial oxygenation, and ventilation/perfusion mismatching.

5. As people age, they are at greater risk for developing postoperative complications such as atelectasis and pneumonia. This is due to a number of physiologic changes associated with the aging process. With advancing age, lung volumes and mechanics demonstrate a progressive decline in pulmonary function. The elastic recoil of the lung decreases and there is progressive stiffening of the chest wall. Changes in the musculoskeletal system—such as gradual loss of bone and muscle mass, as well as general wear and tear on joints—contribute to activity intolerance and impaired mobility. Decreases in lung volume and immobility are two important factors increasing the risk of postoperative complications.

6.

Spirometric Indicators of Risk and High Risk for Postoperative Pulmonary Complications*

Measurement	At Risk	At High Risk
FVC	<50% of predicted	<1.5 L
FEV_1	<50% of predicted	<1.0 L
FEV1	<2.0 L	
FEV_1/FVC	<50%	<35%
$FEF_{25\%-75\%}$	<50% of predicted	
MVV		<50% of predicted

*FVC = forced vital capacity; FEV_1 = forced expiratory volume in 1 second; $FEF_{25\%-75\%}$ = forced expiratory flow, midexpiratory phase; MVV = maximal voluntary ventilation.

From Barnes TA: Core textbook of respiratory care practice, ed 2, St. Louis, 1994, Mosby.

7. T
8. T
9. T
10. F
11. T
12. F

Topic 2: Incentive Spirometry

13. The physiologic basis for sustained maximal inspiration maneuvers is that it increases the transpulmonary pressure gradient and helps fully expand alveoli. This maneuver combined with a few-seconds breath hold can prevent and/or treat atelectasis.

14. The indications for incentive spirometry include pulmonary atelectasis, presence of conditions predisposing patients to atelectasis (thoracic surgery, upper abdominal surgery, and surgery in patients with COPD), presence of a restrictive lung defect associated with quadriplegia and/or dysfunctional diaphragm.

15. Contraindications to incentive spirometry include the following cases: patients who cannot be instructed or supervised to assure proper use of the device, patients unable to understand or unwilling to perform sustained maximal inspiration technique, and patients unable to breathe effectively (e.g., vital capacity less than 10 ml/kg, or inspiratory capacity less than about one-third of predicted).

16. The hazards and complications of incentive spirometry are few, especially when the therapy is properly supervised. The hazards and complications include hyperventilation and respiratory alkalosis, pulmonary barotrauma (emphysematous lungs), hypoxemia (with interruption of therapy), discomfort secondary to inadequate pain control, exacerbation of bronchospasm, and fatigue. In addition, incentive spirometry is ineffective unless closely supervised or performed as ordered. It is inappropriate as sole treatment for major lung collapse or consolidation.

17. There are many advantages to performing preoperative incentive spirometry assessment and teaching. A baseline of lung volumes and capacities can be determined. This will help identify patients at high risk for postoperative complications and help set volume goals after the surgery. Teaching the sustained maximal inspiration maneuver prior to surgery is often easier and it allows time for practice and reinforcement of the technique. It further increases the likelihood that patients will remember and follow instructions postoperatively, when they are usually receiving opioid analgesics which can make patients forgetful. Practice, along with a good understanding of the benefits of incentive spirometry therapy, increases the likelihood of success after surgery.

Keep in mind, however, as healthcare delivery changes, fewer patients are admitted to the hospital prior to surgery. The opportunity for pre-op teaching may diminish. RCPs may be involved in teaching patients in the outpatient setting before their operations.

18. Successful incentive spirometry requires skillful teaching with return demonstration from the patient. Patients must be instructed to inspire slowly and deeply to maximize the distribution of ventilation and to reach the predetermined goal. The goal should be one that requires patient effort, but is attainable so that the patient does not become discouraged. Correct technique will emphasize diaphragmatic breathing at slow inspiratory flows. Each deep breath should be held for 5 to 10 seconds. Patients should perform incentive spirometry at a minimum of 5 to 10 sustained maximal inspiration maneuvers each hour. They should be instructed to rest between deep breaths to avoid hyperventilation.

19. Respiratory care practitioners should set a schedule for return visits to monitor patient use and check technique. Patients often require reinstruction and coaching to perform incentive spirometry effectively, especially if they are receiving postoperative opioid analgesics. Observe patient performance and note pattern of use, including frequency of sessions, number of breaths per session, inspiratory volume or flow goals achieved, success with 3- to 5-second breath hold, and effort/motivation. These parameters, including vital signs, should all be documented. Each day, the patient should be reassessed, and, ideally, the goal should be adjusted upward toward the patient's preoperative or predicted inspiratory capacity.

20. Incentive spirometry outcome assessment demonstrating the absence of or improvement in signs of atelectasis includes evidence of decreasing respiratory rate; resolution of fever; normal pulse rate; absent crackles or presence of or improvement in previously absent or diminished breath sounds; normal chest radiograph; improved arterial oxygen tension and decreased alveolar-arterial oxygen tension gradient, or $P(A-a)O_2$; increased vital capacity and peak expiratory flows; and the return of functional residual capacity or vital capacity to preoperative values in absence of lung resection. The outcome assessment for improved inspiratory muscle performance includes evidence of attainment of preoperative flow and volume levels and increased forced vital capacity.

21. Diagram A is a flow-oriented incentive spirometer. Diagram B is a volume incentive spirometer.

22. To calculate the inspired volume with a flow-oriented incentive spirometer, the following formula is used:

$$V \text{ (liters)} = \frac{V \text{ (cc/second) x time (seconds)}}{1000}$$

For this example, the estimated volume would be 3.6 liters.

23. T
24. T
25. F
26. T
27. T

Topic 3: Intermittent Positive Pressure Breathing

28. IPPB is the application of positive inspiratory pressure as a short-term therapy for spontaneously breathing patients. Instead of the normal negative alveolar pressure gradient causing gas to flow into the lungs, positive pressure at the airway opening creates the gradient and pushes gas into the lungs.

29. IPPB therapy is indicated when there is a need to improve lung expansion (e.g., atelectasis not responsive to other therapies, inability to clear secretions due to ineffective cough or pathology), there is a need for short-term ventilatory support as an alternative to tracheal intubation, or when there is a need to deliver aerosol medications when other methods have failed.

30. Untreated tension pneumothorax is an absolute contraindication to IPPB. The following are considered relative contraindications to IPPB: intracranial pressure greater than 15 mm Hg, hemodynamic instability, recent facial, oral, or skull surgery, tracheoesophageal fistula, recent esophageal surgery, active hemoptysis, nausea, air swallowing, active untreated tuberculosis, radiographic evidence of bleb, and hiccups.

31. Hazards/complications of IPPB include increased airway resistance, barotrauma, pneumothorax, nosocomial infection, hypocapnia, hemoptysis, hyperoxia when oxygen is the gas source, gastric distension, impaction of secretions (associated with inadequately humidified gas mixture), psychologic dependence, impedance of venous return, exacerbation of hypoxemia, hypoventilation, increased mismatch of ventilation and perfusion, air trapping, auto-PEEP, and over-distended alveoli.

32. Baseline assessment of a patient about to receive IPPB therapy should include determination of spontaneous tidal volume, vital capacity, and vital signs. Physical examination of the chest should also be performed.

33. Successful IPPB therapy is evidenced by the following outcome criteria: improved inspiratory or vital capacity, increased FEV_1 or peak flow measurements, improved cough and secretion clearance, improved chest radiograph, improved breath sounds, normalization of arterial blood gases, and favorable patient subjective response.

34. While performing IPPB, the following infection control precautions should be observed: proper handwashing before and after therapy, observance of CDC universal precautions, follow CDC guidelines for preventing the spread of tuberculosis, observe all posted infection control guidelines, use only sterile medications and diluents, change equipment every 24 hours or more often when visibly soiled, reusable equipment should be disinfected between patients, and nebulizer should be rinsed with sterile water and never tap water.

35. The respiratory care practitioner should monitor the patient's respiratory rate, blood pressure, heart rate and rhythm, tidal volume, subjective response to therapy (e.g., discomfort, pain, dyspnea, lightheadedness), sputum production, skin color, mental function, breath sounds, saturation by pulse oximetry, and intracranial pressure in patients for whom ICP is monitored.

36. Performance of IPPB equipment should be monitored by evaluation of machine trigger sensitivity, peak inspiratory pressure, flow setting, FIO_2, inspiratory and expiratory time, and I:E ratio.

37. The general goal of IPPB therapy is to improve the patient's inspired volume during therapy as compared to their spontaneous effort. The AARC Clinical Practice Guideline for IPPB suggests tidal volume during IPPB should be at least 25% greater than the spontaneous volume.

38. T
39. F
40. T
41. T
42. T
43. T
44. T
45. F
46. T
47. F
48. T
49. T
50. T
51. F
52. T

Topic 4: Positive Airway Pressure Breathing

53. Positive airway pressure is a form of treatment designed to increase the transpulmonary pressure gradient and enhance lung expansion. Continuous positive airway pressure (CPAP), expiratory positive airway pressure (EPAP), and positive expiratory pressure (PEP) are all examples.

54. EPAP therapy requires the patient to exhale against a threshold resistor that generates a preset pressure of 10 to 20 cm H_2O. The expiratory pressures generated by the patient are independent of flow. In PEP therapy, the patient exhales against a fixed-orifice flow resistor. Expiratory pressures are dependent on the patient's expiratory flow. When the patient creates higher expiratory flow through the fixed-orifice, the expiratory pressure will increase. Patients are instructed to maintain a pressure between 10 to 20 cm H_2O. CPAP therapy maintains a positive airway pressure throughout both inspiration and expiration. In this way CPAP elevates and maintains high alveolar and airway pressures throughout the full breathing cycle.

55. Indications for positive airway pressure adjuncts include the need to reduce air trapping in asthma and COPD, to aid in mobilization of retained secretions (in cystic fibrosis and chronic bronchitis), to prevent or reverse atelectasis, and to optimize delivery of bronchodilator in patients receiving bronchial hygiene therapy.

56. There are no absolute contraindications to positive airway pressure therapy (CPAP, PEP, and EPAP). The following are the relative contraindications provided by the AARC Clinical Practice Guidelines: patients unable to tolerate the increased work of breathing (asthma, COPD), intracranial pressure (ICP) greater than 20 mm Hg, hemodynamic instability, recent facial, oral or skull surgery or trauma, acute sinusitis, epistaxis, esophageal surgery, active hemoptysis, nausea, known or suspected tympanic membrane rupture or other middle ear pathology.

57. Hazards and complications associated with positive airway pressure adjuncts include the following: increased work of breathing that can lead to hypoventilation and hypercarbia; increased intracranial pressure; cardiovascular compromise; air swallowing, increasing the likelihood of vomiting and aspiration; claustrophobia; skin breakdown and discomfort from the mask; and pulmonary barotrauma.

58. When selecting candidates for positive airway pressure therapy, the following parameters should be assessed to establish need: sputum retention not responsive to spontaneous or directed cough; history of pulmonary problems treated successfully with postural drainage therapy; decreased breath sounds or adventitious sounds suggesting secretions in the airway; change in vital signs, such as increased respiratory rate or tachycardia; abnormal chest radiograph consistent with atelectasis; mucus plugging; infiltrates; and deterioration in arterial blood gas values or oxygen saturation.

59. Assessment of outcome examines those areas targeted for improvement. For example, if sputum retention was the problem, sputum should be evaluated and increased sputum production indicates a positive outcome. Breath sounds should clear or indicate movement of secretions into larger airways. Changes in vital signs toward normal would be a positive outcome. Chest radiographs should be evaluated for resolution or significant improvement in atelectasis and localized infiltrates. As the patient's condition improves, normal oxygenation should return. Patient's subjective response to therapy can also be considered as part of the assessment of outcome.

60. PEP requires a fixed orifice resistor and one-way valves allowing unobstructed inspiration. CPAP requires a threshold resistor with a source of gas flow (e.g., blender, reservoir, or demand valve). EPAP requires a threshold resistor with one-way valve to direct exhaled gas through it. Additional equipment includes transparent mask/mouthpiece and pressure manometer.

61. Monitoring of patients receiving CPAP, EPAP, and PEP therapy would include assessment of vital signs (heart rate and rhythm, respiratory rate, blood pressure), breathing pattern, chest and abdominal excursion, sputum production, mental function, skin color, and breath sounds. When appropriate, pulse oximetry and intracranial pressure monitoring should be performed.

62. T
63. F
64. T
65. F
66. T

Topic 5: Follow-up to Mrs. Howell

67. Following the protocol, this patient can be changed to supervised incentive spirometry twice a day for 48 hours. She should be monitored and coached to continue deep breathing and coughing every hour between visits by the respiratory care practitioner to ensure a pulmonary complication-free recovery. The RCP should collaborate with Mrs. Howell's nurses to assure therapy is performed every hour in the RCP's absence.

68. Although there are no overt signs of postoperative pulmonary complications, the patient's inspiratory volumes should be increasing. The therapist needs to determine the cause of the sustained low lung volumes. Causes may include poor effort, poor understanding of the technique, poor position, and lack of pain control. The patient should be monitored closely and the nurse/physician should be notified of the findings.

69. In this case, Mrs. Howell needs to be evaluated for the secretion management protocol. The incentive spirometry alone is not effective.

70. Mrs. Howell seems to be well on the road to recovery. She no longer needs visits by the respiratory care department but she should be strongly encouraged to work with the incentive spirometer on her own. Nursing should be notified that she is no longer on the respiratory care service and she should be monitored and coached. Chart documentation should be completed.

Posttest Answers

1. d
2. b
3. b
4. c
5. d
6. c
7. b
8. a
9. d
10. a
11. d
12. b
13. d
14. b
15. a
16. b
17. a
18. c
19. c
20. a
21. b
22. c
23. d
24. d
25. a

Unit 5: Physical Assessment

Topic 1: Initial Patient Assessment and History

1. The patient interview is done prior to the actual physical assessment when time and patient condition allows. The interview is important because it allows the respiratory care practitioner the opportunity to (1) determine the patient's perspective concerning his or her illness and (2) develop the medical history. This is the time to establish a professional, open atmosphere between the practitioner and the patient. This type of atmosphere will facilitate information gathering so that changes in the patient's condition and response to treatment can be monitored.

2. Interviewers should remember the following guidelines when conducting patient interviews: address patients using their full names; state the intent of the interview; project your interest in the patient by listening intently and providing nonverbal cues such as nodding your head to signify agreement; provide the patient with privacy; proceed in a nonhurried, professional manner; maintain eye contact as appropriate; question and clarify responses as needed; and adjust the interview to the patient's needs.

3. The chief complaint is the reason the patient is seeking health care.

4. The respiratory care practitioner should gather information about the present illness, including its signs, symptoms, onset, quality, frequency, duration, severity, location, aggravating or alleviating factors, and any associated manifestations.

5. Taking a few seconds to get a general sense of your patient is helpful in determining the acuity and severity of your patient's condition. This will help you determine your course of action and approach to the patient.

6. Sensorium is traditionally evaluated by determining the patient's orientation to time, place, and person. You can also determine how the patient answers questions and whether the patient is forgetful or is able to follow a train of thought.

7. Observing facial expression can provide clues to alertness, pain, anxiety, mental capacity, and mood of the patient.

8. A comprehensive patient history would include the following: today's date, the patient's name, age, sex, occupation, chief complaint, history of present illness, medical history, family history, psychosocial history, and a review of the patient's body systems.

9. The Weed system of patient evaluation reports on four aspects commonly referred to as *SOAP*. The *S* is for the subjective evaluation of the patient. Documentation includes how the patient feels or any complaints offered at the time of the evaluation. *O* refers to the objective findings such as vital signs, breath sounds, peak expiratory flowrate (PEFR), and laboratory data. The *A* is for the assessment of the subjective and objective information. The assessment is where the RCP puts the information together and gives it meaning. *P* refers to the plan of care based on the evaluation of the patient. It refers to the action to be taken based on the findings.

10. F
11. T
12. T
13. F
14. T

Topic 2: Vital Signs

15. The average normal body temperature for adults is 37° C with daily variations of approximately 0.5° C.

16. An elevation in body temperature will increase the body's metabolic rate and, therefore, increase both oxygen consumption and carbon dioxide production. Oxygen consumption and carbon dioxide production increase by 10% for every 1° C rise in body temperature.

17. Patients with hypothermia exhibit slow and shallow breathing and a decreased heart rate because hypothermia reduces oxygen consumption and carbon dioxide production. Therefore, the demand on the heart and lungs is reduced.

18. The normal pulse rate is 60 to 100 beats per minute with a regular rhythm.

19. Pulsus paradoxus is a notable decrease in pulse strength during inhalation. It is exhibited in patients with obstructive lung disease (most notably during asthma attacks) and pericardial tamponade. This finding may be easier to detect while auscultating blood pressure. The Korotkoff sounds will fade in intensity during inspiration, then return to normal with exhalation.

20. The normal resting respiratory rate for adults is 12 to 20 breaths per minute.

21. A slow respiratory rate may be seen in patients who have head injuries or hypothermia. It may also occur as a drug side effect with medications such as narcotics or as a result of certain drug overdoses.

22. The normal adult blood pressure is 95 to 139 mm Hg systolic and 60 to 89 mm Hg diastolic.

23. Hypotension is a blood pressure less than 95/60 mm Hg and is caused by low blood volume, peripheral vasodilatation, and/or left ventricular heart failure.

24. Hypertension is a blood pressure of 140/90 mm Hg or higher. It is most commonly a result of high systemic vascular resistance of unknown cause. Ninety percent of cases are idiopathic.

25. Any of the following can result in falsely high blood pressure measurements: using a blood pressure cuff that is too small (narrow); applying the cuff too tightly; applying the cuff too loosely so that when inflated, the edges act as a tourniquet on the arm; using an inflation pressure that is too high, or holding the pressure in the cuff too long; and not completely deflating the cuff between measurements.

26. F
27. F
28. T
29. T
30. F
31. T
32. T
33. T
34. F
35. T

Topic 3: Chest Physical Assessment

36. A barrel chest is denoted by an increased anteroposterior diameter; a funnel chest is identified by a depression in the lower portion of the sternum; a pigeon chest is characterized by the anterior displacement of the sternum; scoliosis is a lateral curvature of the spine; and kyphosis is an abnormal anteroposterior curvature of the spine.

37. Inspection of a patient generally begins at the patient's head and neck. Facial expression, color of skin and mucous membranes, presence of jugular vein distention, and presence or absence of nasal flaring are all examples of what should be observed. When inspecting the thorax, the respiratory care practitioner should assess thoracic configuration, accessory muscle use, chest symmetry, breathing pattern and effort. The extremities should be inspected for edema, clubbing, nailbed color, and capillary refill.

38. Abdominal paradox is seen when the abdomen sinks inward during inspiration instead of moving outward. It is seen in paralysis or fatigue of the diaphragm.

39. Respiratory alternans is a breathing pattern (seen with fatigue) in which the patient breathes for a period of time with his or her chest muscles and then for a period of time with the diaphragm alone.

40. Palpation is the act of touching the patient to evaluate underlying structure and function. Palpation of the chest is used to evaluate vocal fremitus, estimate chest expansion, locate the placement of the trachea and cardiac impulse, and assess the skin and subcutaneous tissue of the chest.

41. Percussion is the art of systematic tapping on the body to evaluate underlying tissues.

42. Diseases such as pneumonia, tumor, and atelectasis will produce a dull percussion note. Asthma and emphysema (with air trapping) and pneumothorax can produce a hyperresonant percussion note.

43. Some of the common errors made while auscultating the chest include listening over clothing; listening in a noisy room; allowing the tubing to lay against the patient, bed, or other objects; auscultating only a couple of locations (or those that are convenient); and interpreting chest hair sounds as adventitious sounds. Each of these mistakes is easily avoided.

44. Vesicular breath sounds are located in the peripheral areas of the lungs.

Bronchovesicular breath sounds are located around the upper part of the sternum between scapulae.

Bronchial breath sounds are located over the trachea.

45. Crackles are discontinuous sounds; wheezes are continuous sounds.

46. A pleural friction rub is most often described as a grating or creaking sound produced on inspiration, expiration, or both when the pleural surfaces become inflamed.

47. Whispered pectoriloquy is the increased ability to hear whispered words through auscultation. It is especially helpful when assessing patients with small areas of consolidation. The consolidated area transmits the words more clearly as compared to normal lung tissue. In this way, small areas of consolidation can be identified.

48. Stridor is a high-pitched, distinctive upper airway sound. Stridor is heard in croup, epiglottitis, and postextubation edema.

49. Capillary refill is assessed by firmly pressing on a fingernail for a brief period and releasing while observing the color return to the nail bed. Normal capillary refill returns color within 2 to 3 seconds. Slow capillary refill may be a sign of poor cardiac output or decreased digital perfusion.

50. Clubbing is the painless enlargement of the terminal phalanges of the fingers and toes associated with cardiopulmonary disease, most notably cystic fibrosis.

51. F
52. F
53. F
54. T
55. F
56. T
57. F
58. T
59. T
60. T
61. C
62. D
63. E
64. F
65. A
66.

Abnormality	Initial Impression	Inspection	Palpation	Percussion	Auscultation	Possible Causes
Acute airway obstruction	Appears acutely ill	Use of accessory muscles	Reduced expansion	Increased resonance	Expiratory wheezing	Asthma, bronchitis
Chronic airway obstruction	Appears chronically ill	Increased anteroposterior diameter, use of accessory muscles	Reduced expansion	Increased resonance	Diffuse reduction in breath sounds; early inspiratory crackles	Chronic bronchitis, emphysema
Consolidation	May appear acutely ill	Inspiratory lag	Increased fremitus	Dull note	Bronchial breath sounds; crackles	Pneumonia, tumor
Pneumothorax	May appear acutely ill	Unilateral expansion	Decreased fremitus	Increased resonance	Absent breath sounds	Rib fracture, open wound
Pleural effusion	May appear acutely ill	Unilateral expansion	Absent fremitus	Dull note	Absent breath sounds	Congestive heart failure
Local bronchial obstruction	Appears acutely ill	Unilateral expansion	Absent fremitus	Dull note	Absent breath sounds	Mucous plug
Diffuse interstitial fibrosis	Often normal	Rapid shallow breathing	Often normal; increased fremitus	Slight decrease in resonance	Late inspiratory crackles	Chronic exposure to inorganic dust
Acute upper airway obstruction	Appears acutely ill	Labored breathing	Often normal	Often normal	Inspiratory/expiratory stridor	Epiglottitis, croup, foreign body aspiration

From Wilkins RL, Krider SJ, and Sheldon RL, editors: Clinical assessment in respiratory care, ed 3, St. Louis, 1995, Mosby.

Topic 4: Chest Trauma

67. Depending on the size of the pneumothorax and the pulmonary reserve of the patient, signs and symptoms of a pneumothorax will vary. In general, the patient will appear acutely short of breath with an increased respiratory rate. Chest expansion may be reduced, percussion will be hyperresonant, breath sounds distant, and tactile fremitus decreased over the pneumothorax. With a large tension pneumothorax, the trachea and mediastinum can shift away from the affected side. Heart rate and blood pressure will increase initially, but in cases of a tension pneumothorax and decreased venous return, these values will decrease.

68. A tension pneumothorax occurs when air continues to enter the intrapleural space and cannot escape. The pressure builds, and the intrapleural pressure exceeds the atmospheric pressure throughout expiration. The increased pressure can cause the mediastinum to shift away from the affected side. The venae cavae and pericardium can be compressed, resulting in decreased venous return to the heart and reduced cardiac output.

69. A pneumomediastinum is air in the mediastinum. It most often occurs as a result of alveolar rupture, and is seen more commonly in mechanically ventilated newborns. It can also occur as a result of injury to the upper respiratory tract, intrathoracic airways or gastrointestinal tract.

70. A pleural effusion is defined as excess fluid in the pleural space. The fluid can be of many types, such as serous fluid, blood, chyle, and pus.

71. The signs and symptoms of a pleural effusion depend on a number of factors, such as the amount of fluid present in the pleural space, the patient's underlying condition or coexisting disease, and the extent of pulmonary compromise. Common symptoms include dyspnea, chest pain, decreased tactile fremitus, dullness to percussion, and dry, nonproductive cough.

72. Paradoxical chest wall movement is the inward movement of the chest (or segment of the chest) on inspiration and the outward movement on expiration. This occurs when there is an unstable segment with broken ribs. Three or more adjoining ribs fractured in two or more places is known as a flail chest. This segment may move in when negative intrathoracic pressure is generated with inspiration, the opposite movement seen with the stable chest.

73. Subcutaneous emphysema is free air in the subcutaneous tissues. It can be felt as a crackling sensation during chest palpation. Subcutaneous emphysema most commonly results from air escaping from a laceration in the lung or chest wall as a result of trauma or surgery.

74. T
75. F
76. T
77. T
78. T

Topic 5: Chest Drainage

79. The purpose of closed chest drainage is to remove air and/or fluid from the pleural space. A closed chest drainage system acts as an extension of the patient's pleural space.

80. Chest drainage is indicated when the presence of air or fluid in the pleural space is compromising the patient's ability to oxygenate—and when dyspnea, chest pain, and arterial hypoxemia are present. The amount of air and/or fluid resulting in compromise depends on the patient's general condition and pulmonary reserve.

81. The device is a Heimlich valve. It provides one-way evacuation of air from the pleural space when attached to a chest tube. It is especially useful during transport of patients requiring chest drainage and as a tool in emergency situations requiring immediate air evacuation from the chest, such as during cardiac resuscitation complicated by pneumothorax.

82. The water seal functions as a one-way valve, allowing air to exit the pleural space by bubbling through the system, while preventing air from returning to the pleural space.

83. Continuous bubbling in the water seal chamber indicates air is continuously being supplied to the system. This can be seen in patients with a large active pneumothorax or bronchopleural fistula, in patients receiving positive end expiratory pressure (PEEP), and when there is a leak in the chest drainage system. Intermittent bubbling can be seen with cough, positive pressure mechanical breaths, or bearing down (Valsalva's maneuver). Absent bubbling in the water seal chamber usually indicates the air leak has been resolved and the lung is totally reexpanded, but it could indicate an obstruction between the pleural space and chest drainage system.

84. The collection chamber provides an area for fluid to be collected and measured. The nature of the fluid (bright red blood, serosanguineous or serous fluid) and the amount and rate of drainage should be monitored.

85. The suction control chamber regulates the amount of negative pressure applied to the pleural space. Suction hastens the removal of air and fluid from the pleural space and can facilitate the reexpansion of the lung.

86. A: suction control, B: water seal, C: collection.

87. T
88. T
89. F
90. T
91. T

Topic 6: Assessment of the Trauma Patient

92. Start with the *ABC*s. The first priority is to assess the airway. The respiratory care practitioner must quickly determine if the airway is patent or obstructed by evaluating whether air movement is present.

93. When a patient has a partially occluded airway, sound is produced by airflow past the obstruction. The air movement is usually noisy. The patient may also demonstrate an increased effort to move air and to breathe. In this case, tachypnea, tachycardia, suprasternal and intercostal muscle retractions, anxiety, and nasal flaring are present. The hallmark of a totally occluded airway is the absence of sound. The patient can demonstrate extreme effort to move air. The signs include sternal and intercostal retractions, cyanosis, panic, and diaphoresis. A patient in traumatic arrest will not make any respiratory effort.

94. Airway occlusion can be caused by loss of muscle tone; aspiration of food, vomitus or foreign body; swelling of the larynx or internal neck tissue; spasm of the larynx; and bilateral vocal cord paralysis.

95. In trauma patients, the airway should be opened using the jaw thrust/chin lift while maintaining cervical spine immobilization. Suctioning may be needed to remove secretions, vomitus, or debris obstructing the airway. In some cases, the airway is maintained by oral or nasal airway adjuncts, intubation, or cricothyrotomy.

96. Breathing is assessed in the trauma patient much like it is assessed during a routine physical examination. In this case, however, rapid assessment is critical. The clinician must look for emerging respira-

tory complications. First, the respiratory care practitioner determines the presence or absence of breathing. If the patient is not breathing, ventilation must be assisted, using a bag valve device. Airway adjuncts or intubation may be required. When breathing is present, it should be supported with high concentrations of oxygen while respirations are assessed for rate, rhythm, and depth. Breath sounds are evaluated after a brief assessment of airway, breathing, and circulation.

97. When assessing circulation, the respiratory care practitioner must initially evaluate pulse rate and quality to determine if an adequate pulse is present. If not, basic life support and advanced cardiac life support measures should be instituted immediately. Secondary assessment includes blood pressure, skin temperature and color, and capillary refill. Adequate circulation results in normal pulse rate and blood pressure, skin that is warm and dry, and capillary refill within 2 to 3 seconds. Signs of inadequate blood flow include increased heart rate; low blood pressure; cold, clammy skin; and capillary refill time greater than five seconds.

98. Oxygen delivery depends on the quantity of blood flow (cardiac output) and the amount of oxygen carried in the blood (arterial oxygen content). Trauma patients may lose circulating blood volume through hemorrhage, resulting in an absolute hemoglobin deficiency, which will decrease total oxygen content. Cardiac output can be decreased in circulatory failure of shock. Because oxygen delivery depends on both cardiac output and oxygen content, trauma patients are often at risk of tissue hypoxia.

Topic 7: Follow-up to Mr. Donovan

99. Your first action is to alert the nurse in the room and call for help. Immediately begin to ventilate with a bag valve mask device without moving his neck. The patient will need to be assessed for presence of circulation and possible need for cardiac compressions and intubation.

100. An obstructed airway in this patient is of special concern because his neck has not been assessed by a physician and therefore, should not be moved. Mr. Donovan's airway should be opened by a jaw-thrust/chin-lift maneuver. If debris is obstructing the airway, attempt to remove it with suction, but be particularly cautious. His intoxication can make him more likely to vomit as a result of stimulation of the gag reflex with upper airway suctioning. Patients like Mr. Donovan may require intubation or cricothyrotomy to secure an airway.

101. Mentation and urine output have not improved. Oxygen delivery to the tissues may be decreased as a result of low blood volume or shock. Further assessment and treatment of circulation is needed. If the patient has lost a significant amount of blood, a CBC and blood type and cross match should be done. Transfusion may be considered.

Posttest Answers

1. d
2. b
3. a
4. a
5. d
6. d
7. c
8. b
9. b
10. d
11. a
12. a
13. b
14. c
15. a

16. c
17. b
18. b
19. c
20. d
21. b
22. d
23. c
24. d
25. a

Unit 6: Pediatrics

Topic 1: Croup and Epiglottitis

1. (1) Classic croup is an inflammation of the subglottic area due to a viral infection. The most common cause of classic croup is the parainfluenza virus but it also can be caused by respiratory syncytial virus (RSV), influenza viruses and *Mycoplasma pneumoniae*. The classic sign is inspiratory stridor. (2) Spasmodic croup has an unknown etiology; however, an allergic component is likely. With this type of croup, the child presents with stridor and barky cough that abruptly stops, usually after a few hours. (3) Laryngotracheobronchitis, also known as bacterial tracheitis, is an infection of the trachea and larynx. *Staphylococcus aureus*, *Haemophilus influenzae* type B and *Streptococcus pyogenes* are known causes. Although this form of croup is rare, it can result in severe respiratory distress and is considered to be life-threatening.

2. Classic croup is most often seen in children between 6 months and 3 years of age.

3. The clinical presentation of classic croup consists of a history of low-grade fever, coughing, and runny nose for one to two days, followed by the onset of fever, stridor, brassy cough, and hoarseness. The stridor becomes worse with agitation and exertion.

4. Treatment of croup depends on the severity of stridor and respiratory distress. Children who are experiencing stridor during exertion only, and not at rest, can be treated with cool mist at home. If stridor is present at rest, the child is usually hospitalized. Treatment consists of cool mist, often using a "croup tent", and small volume nebulizer delivery of racemic epinephrine. Intubation is considered when the child is experiencing increasing respiratory distress and impending respiratory failure. Bacterial tracheitis is treated with the appropriate antibiotic.

5. Epiglottitis is a bacterial infection of the soft tissues of the larynx. It involves the supraglottic region including the epiglottis, aryepiglottic folds, and arytenoid cartilages.

6. Epiglottitis is caused most commonly by *Haemophilus influenzae* type B, and much less commonly by staphylococci and streptococci. The incidence of epiglottitis is decreasing due to the widespread use of the *H. influenzae* type B (HiB) vaccine.

7. The classic clinical presentation of epiglottitis consists of a child with high fever, anxiety, and muffled voice, who is drooling and leaning forward with his or her head and neck extended. The history consists of a rapid onset of symptoms of sore throat, fever, and coughing for 6 to 8 hours prior to seeking medical attention.

8. Treatment of epiglottis is considered a medical emergency and centers around maintaining the child's airway with an endotracheal or tracheostomy tube. When intubation is attempted, it must be done by an experienced, skilled practitioner, and it is imperative to have a surgeon present, able and ready to perform a tracheotomy in case the airway closes during the intubation attempt. The upper airway infection is treated with an appropriate antibiotic. The artificial airway remains in place for 12 to 48

hours, while the inflamed tissue shrinks in response to the antibiotic therapy. Extubation is considered when the clinical signs such as fever have diminished, and an air leak can be detected around the endotracheal tube. Other care is supportive in nature.

9. Stridor is a sound produced by obstruction of the upper airway. It is described as being a harsh, high-pitched sound and is caused by turbulent gas flow in the upper airway.

10. In airway obstruction, there is a narrowing, or decrease, in the size of the lumen. According to Hagen-Poiseuille's law, the flow of gas is directly proportional to the fourth power of the radius of a tube. Therefore, a small decrease in the radius of the upper airway will result in a profound decrease in the flow of gas through that airway. To maintain a normal flow of gas, a greater transthoracic pressure must be generated, and this increases the work of breathing. In addition, the increased transthoracic pressure created during inspiration increases transmural pressure at the obstruction site, and this can narrow the lumen even more. The child can tire from the increased workload, and respiratory failure may develop.

11. F
12. F
13. F
14. F
15. T
16. T
17. T
18. F
19. T
20. T

Topic 2: Physiologic/Anatomical Pediatric Variations and the Care of the Pediatric Patient

21. The number of mucus glands is the same in the infant and the adult. This means the density of mucus glands is greater in infants and children compared to adult patients. Because a child's airways are shorter and narrower than an adult's, illnesses that produce increased amounts of mucus can compromise children and increase their work of breathing more easily. We are born with approximately 20 to 25 million alveoli. As we grow, the number of alveoli increases through alveolar multiplication to between 300 and 600 million during the first several years of life. After the multiplication period, the alveoli increase in size until the chest wall stops growing. At birth, the thoracic cage is much more compliant compared to the adult thoracic cage. The sternum is cartilaginous at birth, and the ribs are highly compliant. The child's thoracic cage does not offer the same support found in the adult's bony structure. During times of respiratory distress, the sternum and soft tissue between the ribs can be drawn inward during inspiration. Accessory muscles attempt to compensate for the compliant thoracic cage but may be ineffective due to their own immaturity.

22. Pediatric patients are more susceptible to airway obstruction than adults as a result of a number of factors. (1) The relatively small size of the pediatric airway is a great disadvantage. The narrow trachea, bronchi, and bronchioles can be severely compromised by the presence of small amounts of swelling of the mucosal lining which decrease the diameter of the airway. (2) Children are susceptible to respiratory infections such as croup, epiglottitis, and bronchiolitis. (3) When the lower airway is obstructed, the child is less able to handle the compromised condition because collateral ventilation between lung units is ineffective and segmental collapse or atelectasis quickly develops. (4) Pediatric patients have little pulmonary reserve when faced with obstructions in the upper or lower airways. A child's small functional residual capacity provides him with little pulmonary reserve to meet the increased metabolic demands required to maintain adequate ventilation and oxygenation under physiologically stressful conditions.

23. The normal respiratory rate (breaths per minute) for a child 6 months to 1 year is 58–75; 1 to 2 years is 30–40; 3 to 6 years is 19–36; 7 to 10 years is 15–31; and 11 to 14 is 15–26 breaths per minute.

24. The signs and symptoms of increased work of breathing in an infant or child include increased respiratory rate, retractions, nasal flaring, irritability/anxiety, grunting, cyanosis, decreased activity level, poor feeding, lack of activity, and poor sleep quality.

25. Auscultation of the pediatric chest can be a great challenge because breath sounds are easily transmitted from the upper airway or across lung fields, making interpretation of findings more difficult.

26. Infancy (birth to one year) is the stage of trust versus mistrust. Toddlerhood (ages one to three years) is the stage of autonomy versus shame and doubt. In these early stages, it is important to remember to approach the infant or child slowly and calmly while leaving some space between you and them. The parent or caregiver should remain with the infant or child so that the child feels secure. It also may help for the child to hold a familiar personal object for a sense of security. Let these children handle minor equipment such as your stethoscope if it helps them focus or adjust to the situation. Acknowledge positive behavior, and be honest with the child and the parent. Take the time to explain how the procedure will feel, saying, for example, "The mist will feel cool on your face." Take the opportunity to educate the parent.

    Early childhood (ages three to six years) is the stage of initiative versus guilt. Again, your approach should be calm, and you should take time to explain the procedure using simple and concrete terms such as "This device will make a mist that you will be able to see, hear, and feel. Let me show you." Offer limited choices to the child to enhance his or her feelings of control such as "You can take this treatment now, or in ten minutes." Try to enlist the child's help; for example, have them hold the mask to their face or hold your stethoscope for you.

    Middle childhood (ages six to twelve years) is the stage of industry versus inferiority. This age group is beginning to understand simple explanations about their anatomy and body functions. Be direct and honest in your approach. Ask if they have any discomfort or pain.

    Adolescence (twelve to nineteen years of age) is the stage of identity and repudiation versus identity confusion. In this stage, anything that makes them different from their peers, such as an illness, can be considered a major tragedy by them. Psychosomatic complaints and mood swings are common. Adolescents should be provided with the choice of being examined and/or interviewed with or without their parent or guardian present. Be honest, non-judgmental, and never condescending when speaking to an adolescent. Support their body image by reporting normal findings to them. Take the opportunity to educate them and provide them with information about illness prevention. This is a prime age to teach about the hazards of cigarette smoking.

27. F
28. T
29. F
30. T
31. T
32. T
33. T
34. T
35. F
36. T

Topic 3: Aerosol Delivery in the Pediatric Population

37. An MMAD greater than or equal to 5 microns is desirable for delivery of aerosol particles to the upper airway.

38. Indications for cool bland aerosol delivery include laryngotracheobronchitis, subglottic edema, postextubation edema, postoperative management of the upper airway, presence of a bypassed airway, and the need to collect a sputum sample.

39. Indications for bland aerosol therapy include diagnosis of laryngotracheobronchitis or croup, stridor, brassy or croup-like cough, and hoarseness following extubation.

40. Aerosol generators for bland aerosol therapy include the ultrasonic nebulizer, large-volume nebulizer, and the small-volume nebulizer. Application equipment includes the mist tent, hood, mouthpiece, mask, face tent, tracheostomy collar, and T-piece.

41. Hazards/complications of bland aerosol therapy include wheezing and bronchospasm, infection, over-hydration, and patient discomfort.

42. Aerosol particle deposition is influenced by ventilatory rate and depth, airway architecture, and particle size.

43. Racemic epinephrine is given by small volume nebulizer. Children less than three years of age usually are unable to correctly hold and use a mouth-piece/reservoir device. They should take the aerosol treatment by mask. When small children are frightened by the equipment, replacing the mask with something familiar like a decorated paper cup that can be held up to the face may facilitate the delivery of the medication.

44. T
45. T
46. T
47. T
48. T

Topic 4: Follow-up to Alyssa Wilkinson

49. Because Alyssa has stridor at rest, she should be admitted and treated with cool mist and, possibly, supplemental oxygen in a croup tent. Her respiratory rate, oxygen saturation, severity of stridor, air exchange, mental status, activity level, and work of breathing should be assessed every 2 to 4 hours, or more often, as her condition dictates.

50. Intubation is indicated when respiratory failure is imminent, as is the case when a child does not respond to therapy and is becoming exhausted. If arterial blood gases are available, intubation is generally indicated when the $PaCO_2$ value is greater than 70 mm Hg and/or the PaO_2 is less than 70 mm Hg on supplemental oxygen concentrations above 80%. The child should be intubated with an endotracheal tube 1 mm smaller than the age-appropriate diameter to avoid traumatizing the inflamed subglottic tissue.

51. This presentation is a medical emergency since it describes epiglottitis and not a croup syndrome. Since manipulation and/or agitation of the child in this condition can trigger complete airway obstruction, a nonthreatening atmosphere must prevail. There should be no attempts to draw blood, insert an intravenous line, or visualize the laryngeal area until a controlled intubation (with back-up preparation for an emergency tracheostomy) is completed. The intubation is often performed in the operating room, where the patient is given inhalational general anesthesia. Direct laryngoscopy is performed to confirm the diagnosis and to guide intubation.

Posttest Answers

1. b
2. a
3. c

4. a
5. d
6. c
7. d
8. a
9. c
10. d
11. a
12. c
13. d
14. a
15. c
16. b
17. c
18. a
19. d
20. d
21. d
22. a
23. c
24. d
25. a

▬ Unit 7: Noninvasive Monitoring ▬▬▬▬▬▬▬▬

Topic 1: Electrocardiography

1.

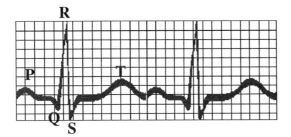

2. The P wave is identified as the first small positive wave, and it represents atrial depolarization. It is followed by the QRS complex, which represents ventricular depolarization. The Q wave is the first negative deflection following the P wave. The R wave is the first positive deflection after the P wave. The S wave is the negative deflection that follows the R wave. The T wave represents ventricular repolarization.

3. The P-R interval represents the length of time required for the atria to depolarize, and the length of time it takes for the sinoatrial (SA) node impulse to travel through the atrioventricular (AV) node to the ventricles. It normally measures 0.12 to 0.20 second.

4. The S-T segment begins with the end of the QRS complex and ends with the onset of the T wave. It represents early repolarization of the right and left ventricles. It is usually not depressed more than 0.5 mm in any lead.

5. The Q-T segment represents the time needed for complete ventricular depolarization and repolarization. It is measured from the start of the QRS complex to the end of the T wave. A prolonged Q-T interval indicates a lengthened relative refractory period which puts the ventricles at risk for life-threatening dysrhythmia.

6. T
7. T
8. T
9. T
10. T
11. F
12. F
13. F
14. T
15. T
16. B
17. F
18. D
19. G
20. E
21. C
22. H
23. A

Topic 2: Pulse Oximetry

24. Pulse oximeters employ two physical principles of operation—spectrophotometry and photoplethys-mography—to measure arterial oxygen saturation. Spectrophotometry measures the absorption of specific wavelengths of light by oxygenated and deoxygenated hemoglobin. Photoplethysmography uses light to measure pulsating blood flow. Combining this technology permits the continuous measurement of arterial saturation and pulse rate.

25. The shape of the oxyhemoglobin curve is important to the relationship between arterial saturation (SaO_2) and the patient's arterial partial pressure of oxygen (PaO_2). The upper portion of the curve becomes flat, so very large changes in PaO_2 result in very small changes in SaO_2. Clinically, this means significant changes can occur in a patient's PaO_2 that may not be reflected by the pulse oximeter. The PaO_2 could fall from 100 mm Hg to 60 mm Hg, and the hemoglobin would still be 90% saturated with oxygen. The steep portion of the curve becomes more linear, and changes in arterial saturation more directly reflect changes in PaO_2. In addition, conditions such as changes in pH, $PaCO_2$, and body temperature will shift the oxyhemoglobin dissociation curve to the right or left. These shifts change the relationship between PaO_2 and SaO_2 and can result in a different saturation for a given PaO_2. A patient's pH, $PaCO_2$, and body temperature must all be considered when evaluating pulse oximetry results.

26. The AARC Clinical Practice Guidelines state the indications for pulse oximetry include the need to monitor the adequacy of arterial oxyhemoglobin saturation, the need to quantitate the response of arterial oxyhemoglobin saturation to therapeutic intervention or to a diagnostic procedure, and the need to comply with mandated regulations or recommendations by authoritative groups.

27. Relative contraindications include the presence of abnormal hemoglobin and the need for ongoing measurement of pH, $PaCO_2$, and total hemoglobin.

28. The accuracy of the pulse oximeter depends on a number of factors. First, the device must be able to detect pulsatile flow to operate. Therefore, low perfusion states or irregular cardiac rhythms may interfere with the ability to obtain adequate measurements. The pulse rate indicated by the pulse oximeter should be verified by the electrocardiographic monitor or by taking the patient's pulse. Abnormal hemoglobin (such as carboxyhemoglobin and methemoglobin) and intravascular dyes can interfere with light absorption and result in inaccurate SpO_2 values. Motion artifact can interfere with the ability of the device to accurately detect pulsatile blood flow, hampering readings. Skin pigmentation can affect the accuracy of measurements by shunting the light away from the photodetector. Greater inaccuracy has been noted in people with dark pigmentation. External factors such as nail polish and nail coverings when using a finger probe and exposure of the measuring probe to ambient

light can interfere with proper function. Pulse oximeters have been shown to be unable to detect saturations below 83% with the same degree of accuracy and precision seen at higher saturations. Finally, as stated earlier, pulse oximeters cannot quantitate the degree of hyperoxemia present. The accuracy of pulse oximeters has been reported to be ± 4%.

29. Pulse oximeter readings (SpO_2) should be initially validated by comparing the readings to those obtained by direct measurement of arterial saturation (SaO_2). The SpO_2 readings can then be periodically reevaluated, depending on the patient's condition. The pulse rate displayed by the pulse oximeter should be compared to that of the patient's counted palpable pulse or a value determined by electrocardiographic monitoring of the patient.

30. F
31. T
32. T
33. T
34. F
35. T
36. F
37. T
38. T
39. F

Topic 3: Capnography

40. The term capnometry refers to the measurement of exhaled carbon dioxide, and capnography generally refers to the graphic display of carbon dioxide measurements during the entire ventilatory cycle. The terms capnometry and capnography are often considered to be synonymous.

41. Gas analysis for carbon dioxide is performed by infrared absorption, mass spectrometry, Raman scattering, or photoacoustic spectra technology. The most common method is the infrared analysis.

42. Gases for analysis of carbon dioxide levels are collected/analyzed using either mainstream or sidestream technology. Mainstream sampling is performed between the endotracheal tube and the ventilatory circuit. In the case of mainstream devices, the patient's exhaled gases pass directly by the carbon dioxide sensor. Sidestream technology uses a sampling port to pump gas away from the patient circuit to a sample chamber located within the device.

43. Advantages of the mainstream capnograph include fast response time, real-time readings, and no sample removal that can reduce tidal volume measurement. Advantages of the sidestream capnograph include lack of a bulky device at the airway, ability to measure N_2O, use on nonintubated patients, and disposable sample lines.

44. When evaluating a capnogram, the height, contour, baseline, frequency, and rhythm should be assessed. The height of the tracing will indicate the end-tidal CO_2 value. The contour of a normal capnogram has a clear CO_2 plateau that is 2 to 5 mm Hg below $PaCO_2$. The baseline of the capnogram indicates the inspired CO_2 level, which should be zero. An elevated baseline indicates rebreathing of CO_2. Frequency and rhythm reflect patient/ventilator activity.

45. The gradient between $PaCO_2$ and $PEtCO_2$ [$P(a\text{-}et)CO_2$] is usually less than 5 mm Hg.

46. End-tidal carbon dioxide levels are effected by alterations in the ventilation/perfusion ($\dot{V}/\dot{Q}$) relationship. Conditions of high ventilation and low perfusion (high $\dot{V}/\dot{Q}$) are deadspace-producing disorders which result in the alveolar carbon dioxide level approaching the inspired carbon dioxide level. This leads to a $PEtCO_2$ value that is less than the $PaCO_2$ and a widening of the [$P(a\text{-}et)CO_2$] gradient. If the $\dot{V}/\dot{Q}$ decreases, as is seen in decreases in ventilation, alveolar carbon dioxide levels rise toward mixed venous carbon dioxide levels.

47. Clinical uses of capnography include the following: to evaluate exhaled CO_2 levels to manage patients on mechanical ventilators; to monitor intentional hyperventilation; to detect ventilator disconnects; to assess of weaning; during cardiopulmonary resuscitation, to monitor the quantity of cardiac output through the pulmonary system; and to detect endotracheal tube placement following intubation.

48. Capnography can be very helpful in detecting inadvertent esophageal intubation. Suspect this condition when the $PEtCO_2$ values do not rise to normal levels immediately after tube placement or when values drop significantly after several breaths. With disposable units, $PEtCO_2$ values are represented by color changes.

49. T
50. T
51. T
52. F
53. T
54. F
55. T
56. T
57. T
58. T
59. E
60. F
61. D
62. G
63. C
64. B
65. A

Topic 4: Follow-up to Beatrice Reilly

66. In this case, both sodium bicarbonate administration and seizure activity have the potential to increase the production of carbon dioxide, and therefore increase the delivery of carbon dioxide to the lungs. Increased $PEtCO_2$ would be expected.

67. Changes in cardiac conduction, a blunted hypoxic drive, and respiratory depression are common in tricyclic poisonings. The capnogram indicated a trend of hypoventilation following normal ventilation. An arterial blood gas should be drawn, and institution of mechanical ventilation should be considered.

68. Beatrice Reilly is still a candidate for continuous pulse oximetry monitoring because her SpO_2 is not stable at this time. She continues to experience seizures with desaturation, and therefore should remain on continuous saturation monitoring and be reevaluated in 24 hours. The pulse oximeter probe should be changed from a fingertip to earlobe probe to reduce the risk of motion artifact during seizures affecting SpO_2 readings.

69. The change in condition suggests the possibility of aspiration pneumonia or ARDS. An arterial blood gas should be drawn, oxygen concentrations increased, and the need for mechanical ventilation considered. At this point she will require close monitoring and aggressive respiratory care.

70. The tracing indicates a disconnect episode from the mechanical ventilator with subsequent reestablishment of mechanical ventilation. This is evidenced by the sudden drop to zero at the time of disconnect, followed by an increased $PEtCO_2$ for a short period of time, and then a normal CO_2 trend.

Posttest Answers

1. a
2. b
3. c
4. b
5. c
6. a
7. b
8. a
9. c
10. d
11. b
12. d
13. c
14. a
15. b
16. c
17. d
18. a
19. b
20. d
21. b
22. d
23. d
24. b
25. a

Unit 8: Mechanical Ventilation

Topic 1: Mechanical Ventilation

1. Mechanical ventilation provides support of the patient that is classified as either full or partial. Full ventilatory support uses a mode of ventilation that provides the patient's full minute ventilation. In full ventilatory support, the ventilator performs all of the work of breathing. Partial ventilatory support uses a mode of ventilation that allows the patient to provide some or all of the minute ventilation. The choice of full or partial ventilatory support is determined by the patient's underlying pathophysiology. For example, patients with hypercapnic respiratory failure or ventilatory muscle weakness/fatigue require full ventilatory support. Patients with pure hypoxemic respiratory failure are treated with partial ventilatory support modes that provide continuous distending pressure.

2. CMV (controlled mechanical ventilation) is a mode of full ventilatory support in which the patient receives a preset number of breaths per minute with a preset tidal volume. A/C (assist/control) is a mode of ventilation that provides a preset number of breaths at a preset tidal volume. In addition, with A/C ventilation, the patient may trigger spontaneous breaths at the preset tidal volume. SIMV is synchronized intermittent mandatory ventilation. With this mode of ventilation, the patient is guaranteed a preset number of breaths at a preset rate. Patients may initiate spontaneous breaths at their own tidal volumes between the mandatory breaths. PSV (pressure support ventilation) is a mode of mechanical ventilation in which the patient's spontaneous breath is augmented by the delivery of a preset pressure limited breath. PCV (pressure control ventilation) provides a preset respiratory rate, and every breath is augmented at a preset pressure limit. MMV (mandatory minute ventilation) is a mode of ventilation designed for weaning from mechanical ventilation. The patient is guaranteed a minimum minute ventilation, and when the desired minute ventilation is not achieved, the ventilator provides positive pressure machine breaths at a preset tidal volume. APRV (airway pressure release ventilation) is a mode of ventilation in which the patient breathes spontaneously at a positive baseline

pressure that is periodically released to a lower pressure level. BiPAP® is a spontaneous breath mode of ventilatory support which allows separate regulation of the inspiratory and expiratory pressures.

3. According to Susan Pilbeam, mechanical ventilation is indicated for the following conditions: apnea or absence of breathing when reversible disease is present; acute respiratory failure; impending respiratory failure; severe hypoxemia attributed to increased work of breathing or an ineffective breathing pattern. A number of indicators are used to assist in the decision to initiate mechanical ventilation. These measurements are outlined in *Egan's Fundamentals of Respiratory Care*, Chapter 29.

4. Tidal volume, less than 5 ml/kg
   Vital capacity, less than 10 ml/kg
   Respiratory rate, greater than 35 breaths/min
   Maximum inspiratory pressure, less than 20 cm H_2O
   $PaCO_2$, greater than 50 mm Hg
   PaO_2, less than 50 mm Hg (room air), less than 70 mm Hg (oxygen)
   Arterial/alveolar PO_2 ratio (PaO_2/PAO_2), less than 0.15

5. High minute ventilation is set 10% to 15% above the targeted minute volume; low minute ventilation is set 10% to 15% below the targeted minute volume; high tidal volume is set 10% to 15% above the tidal volume; low tidal volume is set 10% to 15% below the targeted tidal volume; high inspiratory pressure limit is set 10 to 15 cm H_2O above the average peak airway pressure; low inspiratory pressure is set 5 to 10 cm H_2O below the average peak airway pressure; low PEEP/CPAP is set 3 to 5 cm H_2O less than the PEEP or CPAP level; and FIO_2 alarm should be set 5% above and below the FIO_2 setting.

6. The initial assessment of a patient on mechanical ventilation should include measurement of vital signs, auscultation of the chest to verify bilateral ventilation, assessment of patient's appearance and level of consciousness, verification of endotracheal tube position, patency and cuff pressure, a complete ventilator check, and arterial blood gas analysis.

7. Goals of mechanical ventilation include support or manipulation of gas exchange values such as PaO_2, $PaCO_2$, and pH, improvement of lung volumes, and the reduction or manipulation of the patient's work of breathing.

8. Tidal volume for volume-cycled ventilation is usually calculated from 10 to 15 ml/kg of ideal body weight. The decision to use a tidal volume at 10, 12, or 15 ml/kg depends on factors such as disease, other ventilator settings such as PEEP, and the patient's clinical condition. Ideal body weight formula for male patients is 106 + 6 x (height in inches − 60). The ideal body weight formula for female patients is 105 + 5 x (height in inches − 60).

9. Minute ventilation is commonly determined using the following formulas:
   Females: 3.5(body surface area)
   Males: 4(body surface area)
   Body surface area is determined using the Radford nomogram. In addition, there are a number of clinical conditions requiring adjustment in the estimated minute ventilation. Minute ventilation should be increased by 5% for every degree Fahrenheit above 99, increased by 9% for every degree Celsius above 37, increased 20% for metabolic acidosis. For patients on volume-cycled ventilation, tidal volumes are usually 10 to 15 ml/kg of ideal body weight with machine rates of 8 to 20/min.

10. flowrate is adjusted to meet the patient's inspiratory demand, minimize the work of breathing, and provide an I:E ratio of 1:2 or less (1:3, 1:4). This most often requires a flowrate of 50 to 80 L/min.

11. The physiologic goals of mechanical ventilation include the following: improve or support gas exchange, reduce the work of breathing, and increase lung volume.

12. The patient's $PaCO_2$ can be changed by making changes in the minute ventilation provided to the patient. In volume ventilation, the minute ventilation is changed by altering the rate or tidal volume set on the ventilator. When the goal is to increase minute ventilation, the rate or tidal volume can be increased. Tidal volume increase is often more efficient because it decreases minute deadspace ventilation. To decrease minute ventilation with volume ventilation, the rate or tidal volume can be decreased. Rate is most commonly lowered; however, tidal volume should be lowered when there are concerns of high ventilating pressure and potential lung injury.

    In pressure-targeted modes such as pressure support or pressure control, minute ventilation is altered by adjusting the pressure differential between peak airway pressure and baseline or PEEP pressure. Changes that increase the pressure differential will increase tidal volume, and changes that lower the pressure differential will lower tidal volume.

    The following formula is often used to determine the minute ventilation needed to correct the $PaCO_2$:

$$\text{new } \dot{V}E = \frac{\text{current } \dot{V}E \text{ X current } PaCO_2}{\text{desired } PaCO_2}$$

13. Oxygenation is adjusted to maintain adequate oxygen delivery to the tissues while making every effort to keep the inspired oxygen concentration at a nontoxic level. Oxygenation is maintained by adjusting either the FIO_2 or PEEP/CPAP level. FIO_2 adjustment is usually successful when the hypoxemia to be treated is due to a low $\dot{V}/\dot{Q}$ ratio. FIO_2 changes are not successful when the problem is physiologic shunting; in this case PEEP/CPAP is needed to improve oxygenation.

14. Sigh breaths are indicated before and after suctioning, during and after bronchoscopy, during chest physical therapy, before and during extubation, when small tidal volumes are used with controlled mechanical ventilation, and during the reexpansion of lung collapse. Sigh volume is usually set at 1.5 to 2 times greater than the tidal volume at rates of 5 to 20/hour.

15.
$$Cs = \frac{\text{volume}}{P_{plateau} - PEEP}$$

$$Cs = \frac{500 \text{ ml}}{35 \text{ cm } H_2O - 5 \text{ cm } H_2O}$$

$Cs = 16$ ml/cm H_2O, which is low.

$$R_{aw} = \frac{\text{peak inspiratory pressure} - \text{plateau pressure}}{\text{flow}}$$

$$R_{aw} = \frac{37 \text{ cm } H_2O - 35 \text{ cm } H_2O}{1 \text{ L/sec.}}$$

$R_{aw} = 2$ cm H_2O/L/second, which is normal.

16. After patients are intubated, breath sounds are assessed to assure adequate ventilation of both lungs, and the tube is secured. A chest radiograph will be taken to confirm proper placement. The size of the tube and level of insertion is documented. Cuff pressure should be set by either the minimal leak or minimal occluding volume technique. Actual cuff pressure should be measured after inflation with one of these techniques. Suction equipment, a manual resuscitation bag, and replacement endotracheal tubes should be at the bedside.

17. F
18. T
19. T
20. F

21. T
22. T
23. F
24. T
25. T
26. F
27. A
28. C
29. B
30. D
31. B

Topic 2: PEEP Therapy

32. The indications for PEEP therapy include the following: refractory hypoxemia; PaO_2 increase of less than 10 mm Hg with FIO_2 increase of 0.20; PaO_2 less than 50 mm Hg on an FIO_2 greater than 0.50, shunt greater than 30%; decreased compliance; and recurrent atelectasis with low FRC.

33. The contraindications to PEEP therapy include the presence of an untreated bronchopleural fistula or pneumothorax and severe unilateral lung disease. Relative contraindications include hypovolemia and elevated intracranial pressures.

34. The beneficial physiologic effects of PEEP include increases in compliance and the FRC, decreases in shunt fraction, and increased PaO_2 for a given FIO_2.

35. The potential detrimental physiologic effects of PEEP include cardiovascular compromise, increased work of breathing, increased incidence of barotrauma, increased pulmonary vascular resistance, increased intracranial pressure, increased dead space ventilation, and decreased renal perfusion.

36. The goal of PEEP therapy is to enhance tissue oxygenation, increase compliance, decrease shunting, and increase the FRC. Initiating PEEP is done carefully to minimize the potential cardiovascular and pulmonary complications. PEEP should be increased in small increments of 3 to 5 cm H_2O per step. Parameters such as blood pressure, cardiac output, peak and plateau pressures, compliance, ABG, shunt fraction, and mixed venous values should be monitored.

37. T
38. T
39. F
40. T
41. T

Topic 3: Pulmonary Edema/Myocardial Infarction/Congestive Heart Failure

42. Pulmonary edema is an excessive amount of fluid in the extravascular system and air spaces of the lungs.

43. The etiology of pulmonary edema can be divided into two categories: cardiogenic and noncardiogenic. Causes of cardiogenic pulmonary edema include arrhythmias, left ventricular failure, myocardial infarction, renal failure, and excessive fluid administration. Causes of noncardiogenic pulmonary edema include Adult Respiratory Distress Syndrome (ARDS), inhalation of toxic agents, pneumonia, and therapeutic radiation of the lungs.

44. The radiologic findings consistent with cardiogenic pulmonary edema include dense fluffy opacities that spread from the hilar region to the periphery. The peripheral portion often remains clear, and this produces the classic "butterfly" distribution. Left ventricular hypertrophy is common and pleural effusion may be seen. Kerley's A and B lines may also be seen.

The typical radiologic findings for noncardiogenic pulmonary edema include areas of fluffy densities that are usually more dense near the hilum. The cardiac silhouette is usually not enlarged, and pleural effusion is usually not present.

45. Patients with pulmonary edema may present with the following clinical manifestations: increased respiratory rate, anxiety, cough, frothy sputum, crackles/wheezing, increased tactile and vocal fremitus, cyanosis, decreased PaO_2 on arterial blood gas analysis, and radiographic findings as described in the answer to question 44.

46. Patients with pulmonary edema usually have hypoxemia that requires the use of supplemental oxygen. The hypoxemia is usually caused by the presence of alveolar fluid, atelectasis, and capillary shunting. The hypoxemia caused by shunting is refractory to oxygen therapy, and additional techniques will be needed such as PEEP/CPAP. Besides improving oxygenation, PEEP/CPAP therapy improves lung compliance, decreases the work of breathing, and decreases vascular congestion. A combination of supplemental oxygen and hyperinflation therapy is commonly required.

47. A myocardial infarction is the cardiac event commonly known as a "heart attack." Necrosis of the myocardium occurs when the myocardium is deprived of oxygen as a result of an obstruction in the blood supply.

48. Severe chest pain is generally the first symptom of acute myocardial infarction. The pain is usually more severe than angina pectoris and is persistent. Victims often describe it as "crushing." Radiation of the pain to the jaw, neck, left arm, back and shoulder is also common. Some individuals experience no pain; this is called a "silent" infarction. Victims may experience nausea, vomiting, or the sensation of unrelenting indigestion. Catecholamine release results in diaphoresis and peripheral vasoconstriction resulting in cool and clammy skin. Physical examination reveals abnormal extra heart sounds (S3, S4) reflecting left ventricular dysfunction. Laboratory data reveal leukocytosis and elevated sedimentation rate consistent with inflammation. Cardiac enzymes such as creatine kinase (CK), lactic dehydrogenase (LDH), and serum glutamic oxaloacetic transaminase (SGOT) are released by myocardial cells and therefore rise in the blood. In addition, a twelve-lead ECG will help localize the affected site through identification of Q waves and changes in ST segment and T waves.

49. Functional changes associated with myocardial infarction include decreased cardiac contractility, altered left ventricular compliance, decreased stroke volume and ejection fraction, increased left ventricular end-diastolic pressure, and sinoatrial node malfunction.

50. Complications associated with myocardial infarction include arrhythmia, left ventricular failure (congestive heart failure), pericarditis, rupture of heart structures (septal rupture), thromboembolism, pulmonary embolism, and sudden death.

51. Congestive heart failure is a broad term denoting conditions in which the pumping capability of the heart is impaired.

52. T
53. T
54. T
55. F
56. T
57. T
58. F
59. T
60. T
61. F

Topic 4: Follow-up to Mrs. Gleason

62. Mrs. Gleason requires adjustment of her ventilator settings to improve her oxygenation. Oxygenation can be adjusted by increasing either the FIO_2 or PEEP/CPAP levels. In this case, PEEP is the better choice because of the physiologic shunting associated with pulmonary edema. In general, FIO_2 is increased in increments of 5% and PEEP in increments of 3 to 5 cm H_2O. Mrs. Gleason's PEEP level would be increased to 6 cm H_2O.

63. Mrs. Gleason requires adjustment of her ventilator settings to improve her ventilation and reduce carbon dioxide levels in the blood. When a patient is receiving volume-controlled ventilation, a change in tidal volume or frequency can correct respiratory acidosis. According to the algorithm, the SIMV rate should be increased by 2 breaths per minute, or the tidal volume should be increased by 100 ml.

64. Mrs. Gleason requires a change in the minute ventilation provided by the mechanical ventilator. In pressure-targeted modes such as pressure control, minute ventilation is usually altered by changing the pressure differential. This is done by increasing or decreasing the pressure limit. In this case we need to increase minute ventilation, so we would increase the pressure limit to increase the tidal volume. Changing the rate also is an option, but it is generally less effective than altering the pressure limit in the pressure control mode.

65. The patient has improved and the ABG results are good. At this point the pressure support level could be decreased.

66. Mrs. Gleason meets the criteria for successful weaning and extubation. Continue to wean from pressure support and extubate.

Posttest Answers

1. c
2. a
3. b
4. c
5. d
6. c
7. b
8. c
9. b
10. b
11. c
12. a
13. c
14. a
15. d
16. d
17. c
18. a
19. b
20. d
21. b
22. d
23. a
24. d
25. a

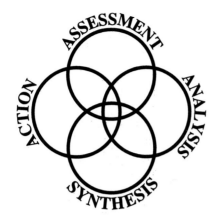

Appendix

Therapist-Driven Protocols

OXYGEN PROTOCOL

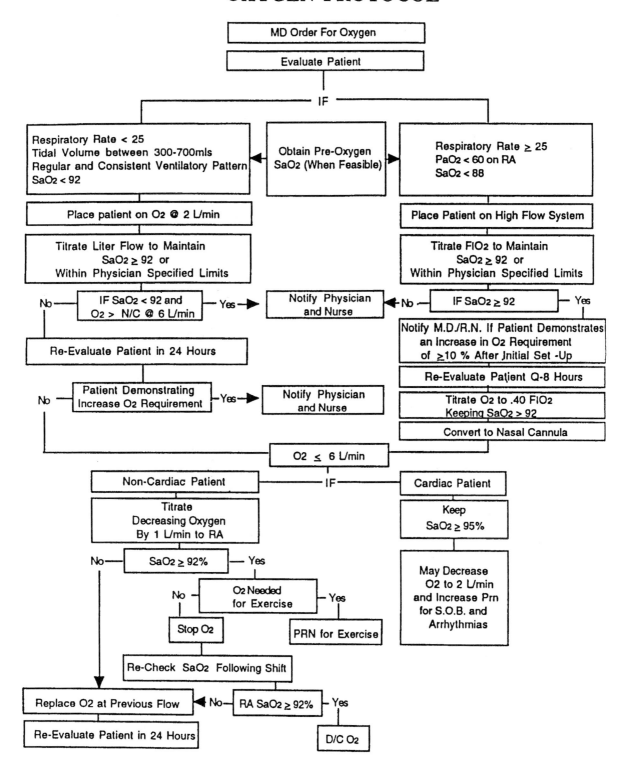

Courtesy of USCD Medical Center, San Diego, California.

RESPIRATORY CARE BRONCHODILATOR ALGORITHM

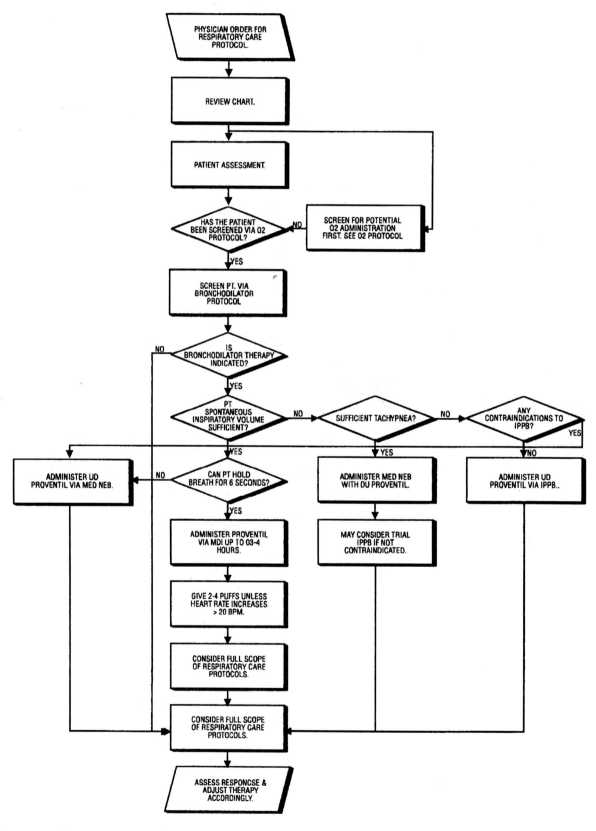

Courtesy of Flower Hospital, Sylvania, Ohio.

RESPIRATORY CARE PULMONARY HYGIENE ALGORITHM

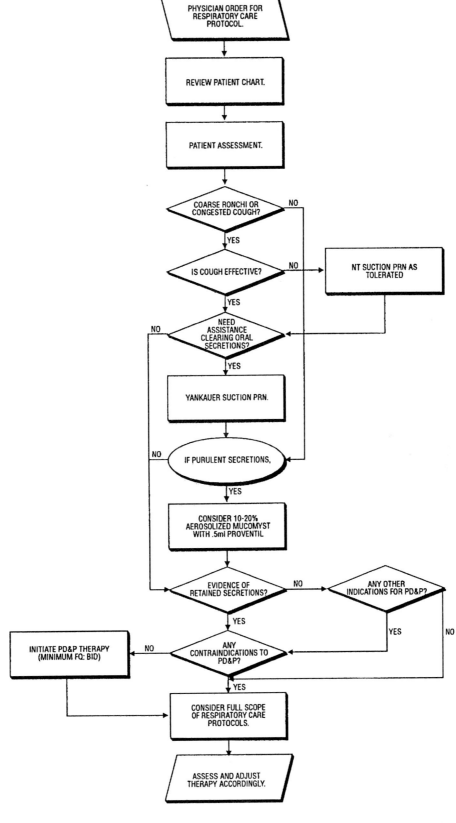

Courtesy of Flower Hospital, Sylvania, Ohio.

PROPHYLAXIS PROTOCOL FOR PULMONARY COMPLICATIONS

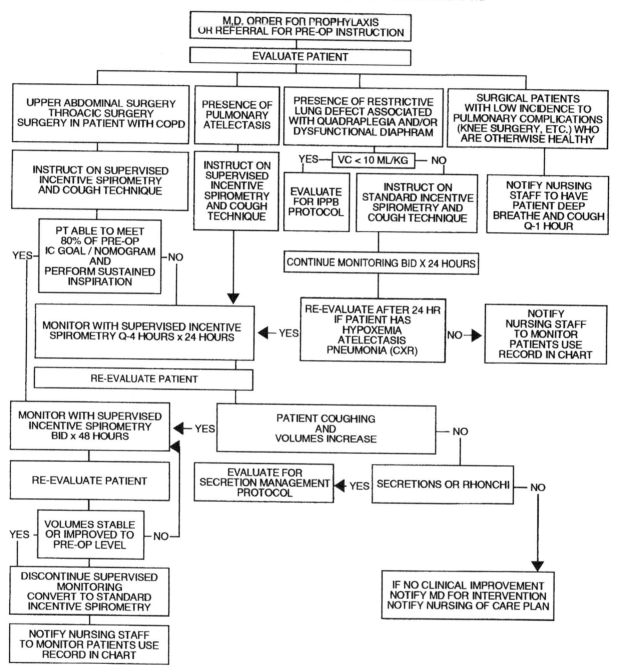

Courtesy of USCD Medical Center, San Diego, California.

TRAUMA PROTOCOL

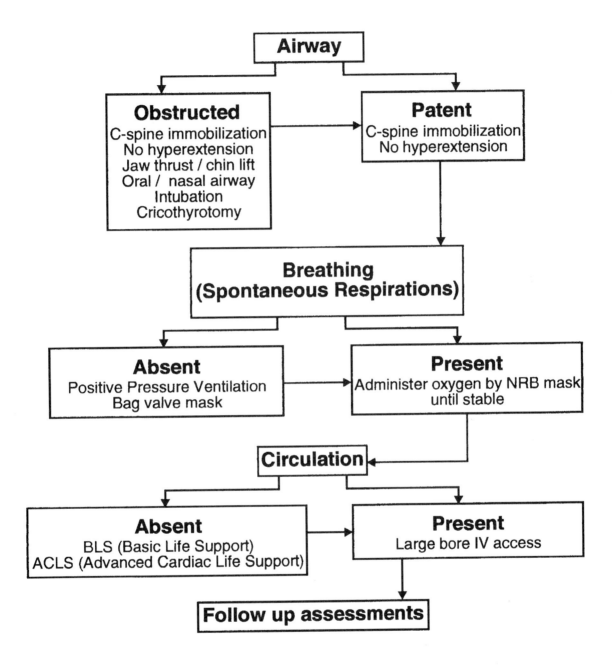

OXIMETRY PROTOCOL

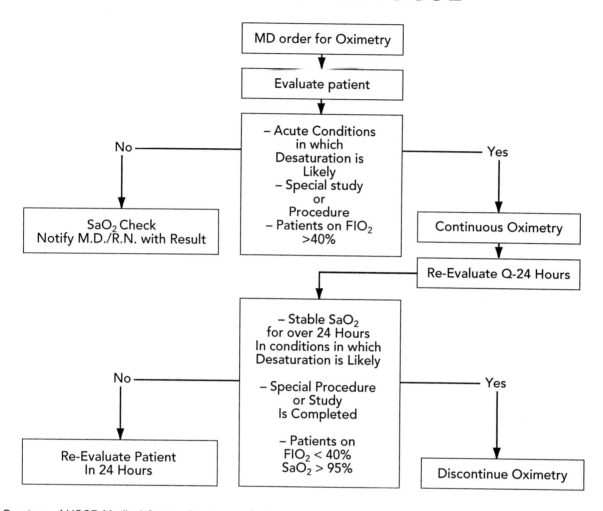

Courtesy of USCD Medical Center, San Diego, California.

MECHANICAL VENTILATION ALGORITHM
(abridged)

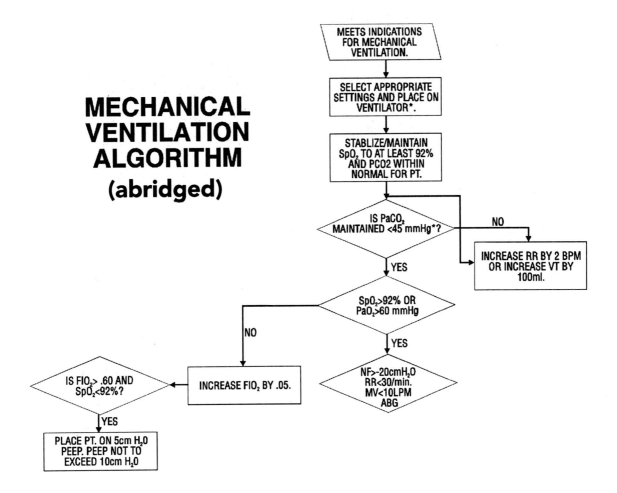

MEETS INDICATIONS FOR MECHANICAL VENTILATION.

SELECT APPROPRIATE SETTINGS AND PLACE ON VENTILATOR*.

STABLIZE/MAINTAIN SpO_2 TO AT LEAST 92% AND PCO2 WITHIN NORMAL FOR PT.

IS $PaCO_2$ MAINTAINED <45 mmHg*?

NO → INCREASE RR BY 2 BPM OR INCREASE VT BY 100ml.

YES

SpO_2>92% OR PaO_2>60 mmHg

NO → INCREASE FIO_2 BY .05.

YES

NF>-20cmH_2O RR<30/min. MV<10LPM ABG

IS FIO_2> .60 AND SpO_2<92%?

YES

PLACE PT. ON 5cm H_2O PEEP. PEEP NOT TO EXCEED 10cm H_2O

Courtesy of Flower Hospital, Sylvania, Ohio.

DATE: July 4		HOSPITAL	Gleason, Alice	ER → CCU 1
VENT. DAY #: 1		PULMONARY SERVICES	7651218	
PRIMARY DR. (NAME) Roche		VENTILATION FLOW SHEET		
PUL. DR. (NAME)				

| DIAGNOSIS: ml | | | |
| OBJECTIVES: vent until stabilized | | | |

	TYPE: 7200	SIZE: 7.5	CM: 23
AIRWAY ACCESS: DATE & TIME OF PLACEMENT: 7/4 1130			
SEDATION:	MUSCLE RELAXANT:		

			TIME	1200	1400					REPORT ON VITAL SIGNS, BREATH SOUNDS, EKG, NEURO STATUS, MEDICATIONS, X-RAYS AND ANY OTHER PERTINENT INFORMATION.
VENTILATOR ORDERS		MODE		SIMV	SIMV					
		VT	ml	750	750					Intub in ED s/p MI.
		f	min	10	10					Neg pulm hx, non-smoker.
		FIO₂	%	40%	40%					Lungs clear, equal BS
		PEEP	cm h₂o	3	3					CXR: WNL ET 3 cm ↑ carina
		PRESS. SUPP.	cm h₂o	0	0					
		AEROSOL MEDICATION		—	—					
ALARMS		HIGH PRESS.	cm h₂o	45	45					HR 84 BP 120/76
		LOW VOLUME	ml	600	600					pulse ox 98% w/ ABG 97%
		LOW VE	L/min	6.0	6.0					1230 hrs ———————— SW RRT
VENTILATOR CHECKS		VT	ml	750	730					
		f	min	10	10					
		VE	L	7.5	7.3					
		PK. PRESS.	cm h₂o	30	32					
		PK. FLOW	L/min	40	40					
		COMP	L/cm h₂o	30	30					
		FIO₂	%	40	40					
		TEMP	°C	37	37					
		PEEP	cm h₂o	3	3					
WEANING PARAMETERS		VT	ml	no	no					
		FVC	L							
		NIF	cm h₂o							
		IMV / SPONT. f	%							
		VD / VT	%							
		COMP	L/cm h₂o							
		f	min							
		VE	L							
ARTERIAL BLOOD GASES		TIME		1230						
		Ph		7.43						
		PaCO₂	mmHg	37						
		PaO₂	mmHg	98						
		SaO₂	%	97%						
		HCO₃	mEq	25						
		THERAPIST INITIALS								

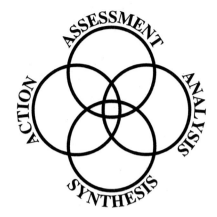

Bibliography

Comprehensive Bibliography

Alfaro-LeFevere R, Blicharz ME, Flynn NM, and Boyer MJ: Drug handbook: a nursing process approach, Redwood City, CA, 1992, Addison Wesley.

American Association for Respiratory Care: Aerosol consensus statement, Resp Care 36:916-921, 1991.

American Association for Respiratory Care: Clinical practice guideline: bland aerosol administration, Resp Care 38:1196-1200, 1993.

American Association for Respiratory Care: Clinical practice guideline: capnography/capnometry during mechanical ventilation, Resp Care 40:1321-1324, 1995.

American Association for Respiratory Care: Clinical practice guideline: delivery of aerosols to the upper airway, Resp Care 39:803-807, 1994.

American Association for Respiratory Care: Clinical practice guideline: incentive spirometry, Resp Care 36:1402-1405, 1991.

American Association for Respiratory Care: Clinical practice guideline: intermittent positive pressure breathing, Resp Care 38:1189-1195, 1993.

American Association for Respiratory Care: Clinical practice guideline: oxygen therapy in the acute care hospital, Resp Care 36:1410-1413, 1991.

American Association for Respiratory Care: Clinical practice guideline: patient-ventilator system checks, Resp Care 37:882-886, 1992.

American Association for Respiratory Care: Clinical practice guideline: postural drainage therapy, Resp Care 36:1418-1426, 1991.

American Association for Respiratory Care: Clinical practice guideline: pulse oximetry, Resp Care 36:1406-1409, 1991.

American Association for Respiratory Care: Clinical practice guideline: selection of aerosol delivery device, Resp Care 37:891-897, 1992.

American Association for Respiratory Care: Clinical practice guideline: selection of an aerosol delivery device for neonatal and pediatric patients, Resp Care 40:1325-1335, 1995.

American Association for Respiratory Care: Clinical practice guideline: use of positive airway pressure adjuncts to bronchial hygiene therapy, Resp Care 38:516-521, 1993.

American College of Chest Physicians: National Heart, Lung, and Blood Institute: National conference on oxygen therapy, Resp Care 29:922-935, 1984.

Barkin RM: Pediatric respiratory emergencies. Emerg Care Q 5:71-78, 1989.

Barnes TA: Core textbook of respiratory care practice, ed 2, St. Louis, 1994, Mosby.

Burton GG and Tietsort JA: Therapist-driven respiratory care protocols (TDP): a practitioner's guide, Torrance, CA, 1993, Academy Medical Systems.

Burton GG, Hodgkin JE, and Ward JJ, editors: Respiratory care: a guide to clinical practice, ed 3, Philadelphia, 1991, JB Lippincott.

Carroll P: Chest tubes made easy, RN 58:46-56, 1995.

Carroll PF: Chest tubes and pleural drainage, AARC Individual Independent Study Package, Dallas, 1992, AARC.

Cherniack RM and Cherniack L: Respiration in health and disease, ed 3, Philadelphia, 1983, WB Saunders.

Dershewitz RA, editor: Ambulatory pediatric care, ed 2, Philadelphia, 1993, JB Lippincott.

DesJardins T and Burton GG: Clinical manifestations and assessment of respiratory disease, ed 3, St. Louis, 1995, Mosby.

Dettenmeier PA: Pulmonary nursing care, St. Louis, 1992, Mosby.

Egan DF: Fundamentals of respiratory therapy, ed 2, St. Louis, 1973, Mosby.

Eubanks DH and Bone RC: Comprehensive respiratory care: a learning system, ed 2, St. Louis, 1990, Mosby.

Frownfelter DL: Chest physical therapy and pulmonary rehabilitation: an interdisciplinary approach, ed 2, St. Louis, 1987, Mosby.

Giordano SP: Aerosol therapy: the hard questions. Resp Care 36:914 -915, 1991.

Gordon PA, Norton JM, and Merrell R: Refining chest tube management: analysis of the state of practice. DCCN 14:6-12, 1995.

Gross SB: Current challenges, concepts, and controversies in chest tube management. AACN Clin Issues Crit Care Nurs 4:260-275, 1993.

Haley K, editor: Emergency nursing pediatric course (provider) manual, Chicago, 1993, Emergency Nurses Association.

Haley K and Baker P, editors: Emergency nursing pediatric course instructor manual, Chicago, 1993, Emergency Nurses Association.

Hathaway WE and Groothuis JR, editors: Current pediatric diagnosis and treatment, ed 10, Norwalk, CT, 1991, Appleton and Lange.

Hess D: Clinical practice guidelines: why, whence, and whither? Resp Care 40:1264-1268, 1995.

Hess D: Reflections on unanswered questions about aerosol therapy delivery techniques. Resp Care 33:19-20, 1988.

Hess D: The AARC clinical practice guidelines, Resp Care 31:1398-1401, 1991.

Jacobs J: How are we doing with operational restructuring and therapist-driven protocols? AARC Times 18:66-69, 1994.

Kacmarek RM: In-hospital O_2 therapy. In Kacmarek RM and Stoller J, editors: *Current respiratory care*, Toronto, 1988, BC Decker.

Kacmarek RM and Hess D: The interface between patient and aerosol generator. Resp Care 36:952-973, 1991.

Keen JH, Baird MS, and Allen JH: Mosby's critical care and emergency drug reference, St. Louis, 1994, Mosby.

Keough V and McNamara P: Case review: a 27-year-old with a tricyclic overdose, J Emerg Nurs 19:382-384, 1993.

Koff PB: Neonatal and pediatric respiratory care, ed 2, St. Louis, 1993, Mosby.

Krueger K: More on management of patient with tricyclic overdose [letter to the editor], J Emerg Nurs 20:173-174, 1994.

Lane EE and Walker JF: Clinical arterial blood gas analysis, St. Louis, 1987, Mosby.

Maas M, Buckwalter KC, and Hardy M: Nursing diagnoses and interventions for the elderly, Redwood City, CA, 1991, Addison-Wesley.

Martin DE and Youtsey JW: Respiratory anatomy and physiology, St. Louis, 1988, Mosby.

McCance KL and Huether SE: Pathophysiology: the biologic basis for disease in adults and children, ed 2, St. Louis, 1994, Mosby.

McPherson SP: Respiratory care equipment, ed 5, St. Louis, 1995, Mosby.

Meltzer LE, Pinneo R, and Kitchell JR: Intensive coronary care: a manual for nurses, Bowie, MD, 1970, The Charles Press.

National Board for Respiratory Care: NBRC '94 examination statistics, NBRC Horizons, March-April: 6-7, 1995.

National Heart, Lung, and Blood Institute: Global initiative for asthma, Bethesda, MD, 1995, Publication number 95-3659, National Institutes of Health.

National Heart, Lung, and Blood Institute: Guidelines for the diagnosis and management of asthma, Bethesda, MD, 1991, Publication number 91-3042, National Institutes of Health.

Nellcor Incorporated: Advanced concepts in capnography, Hayward, CA, 1988, Author.

Nursing 95: Drug handbook, Springhouse, PA, 1995, Springhouse Corporation.

Nursing 96: Drug handbook, Springhouse, PA, 1996, Springhouse Corporation.

Phipps WJ, Long BC, Woods NF, and Cassmeyer VL, editors: Medical-surgical nursing: concepts and clinical practice, ed 4, St. Louis, 1991, Mosby.

Pilbeam SP: Mechanical ventilation: physiological and clinical applications, ed 2, St. Louis, 1992, Mosby.

Poisindex® editorial staff: Toxicologic management: antidepressants, tricyclic, Poisindex®, vol 86, Denver, 1995, Micromedix, Inc.

Price SA and Wilson LM: Pathophysiology: clinical concepts of disease processes, ed 4, St. Louis, 1992, Mosby.

Rau JL: Delivery of aerosolized drugs to neonatal and pediatric patients. Resp Care 36:514-545, 1991.

Rau JL: Respiratory care pharmacology, ed 4, St. Louis, 1994, Mosby.

Rea R, editor: Trauma nursing core course (provider) manual, ed 3, Chicago, 1991, Emergency Nurses Association.

Scanlan CL, Spearman CB, and Sheldon RL, editors: Egan's fundamentals of respiratory care, ed 6, St. Louis, 1995, Mosby.

Schmitz BD and Shapiro BA: Capnography, Respiratory Care Clinics of North America 1:107-117, 1995.

Shapiro BA, Peruzzi WT, and Templin R: Clinical application of blood gases, ed 5, St. Louis, 1994, Mosby.

Sheehy SB: Emergency nursing principles and practice, ed 3, St. Louis, 1992, Mosby.

Sheehy SB: Manual of emergency care, ed 3, St. Louis, 1990, Mosby.

Sly RM: Aerosol therapy in children, Resp Care 36:994-1007, 1991.

Smith J: Big differences in little people, Am J Nurs 88:459-462, 1988.

Society of Critical Care Medicine Task Force on Guidelines: Guidelines for standards of care for patients with acute respiratory failure on mechanical ventilatory support, Crit Care Med 19:275-278, 1991.

Stoller JK: Why therapist-driven protocols? a balanced view, Resp Care 39:706-707, 1994.

Taliaferro E: Disease and trauma monographs for acute care: pneumothorax, Emergindex®, vol 86, Denver, 1995, Micromedix, Inc.

Turner J, McDonald GJ, and Larter NL: Handbook of adult and pediatric respiratory home care, St. Louis, 1994, Mosby.

Urban NA, Greenlee KK, Krumberger JM, and Winkelman C: Guidelines for critical care nursing, St. Louis, 1995, Mosby.

Wilkins RL, Krider SJ, and Sheldon RL, editors: Clinical assessment in respiratory care, ed 3, St. Louis, 1995, Mosby.

Wong DL: Whaley and Wong's nursing care of infants and children, ed 5, St. Louis, 1994, Mosby.

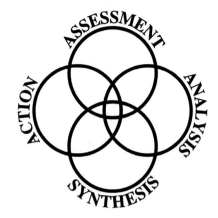

Glossary

Glossary

accessory muscles of respiration additional or reinforcing muscles of the back, neck, and abdomen that play a more prominent role in respiration during exercise or breathing disorder.

acyanotic absence of cyanosis.

adrenergic bronchodilator agent causing stimulation of the sympathetic nervous system.

adult respiratory distress syndrome (ARDS) a pattern of clinical, physiologic, and pathologic features characterizing the lung's response to a variety of injuries and resulting in diffuse damage to the alveolar-capillary membrane; clinically characterized by refractory hypoxemia, decreased lung compliance, and an increased work of breathing.

aerosol a suspension of solid or liquid particles in a gas.

algorithm a predetermined group of directions to solve a problem in a finite number of steps.

American Association for Respiratory Care (AARC) the primary voluntary professional organization for respiratory care practitioners.

analgesia absence of sensibility to pain.

arrhythmia variation from the normal heart rhythm.

arterial blood gas (ABG) refers to the sample of arterial blood or the results of measurement of the partial pressure of oxygen and carbon dioxide, pH, bicarbonate, and oxygen saturation levels; used to assess the adequacy of oxygenation and ventilation.

asthma a respiratory disorder characterized by recurring episodes of paroxysmal dyspnea and wheezing on expiration caused by constriction of the bronchi, coughing, and viscous mucoid bronchial secretions.

aspiration pneumonia inflammation of the lung parenchyma as a result of the inspiration into the lungs of a foreign material such as vomitus.

atelectasis an abnormal condition characterized by the collapse of lung tissue that prevents exchange of carbon dioxide and oxygen with the pulmonary capillary blood.

auscultation the act of listening for sounds within the body to evaluate the condition of organs such as the heart and lungs.

blood pressure the pressure exerted by the circulating volume on the walls of the arteries, veins, and chambers of the heart.

bronchial breath sounds also known as tubular; abnormal breath sounds in which expiration and inspiration produce loud, high-pitched sounds that are equal in duration; can be heard over consolidated lung parenchyma.

bronchodilator a substance, especially a drug, that relaxes contractions of the smooth muscle of the bronchioles to improve ventilation of the lungs.

bundle of His also called the atrioventricular bundle, a band of cardiac muscle fibers connecting the atria with the ventricles and providing a conduction pathway.

capillary refill the process of blood returning to a portion of the capillary system after being briefly interrupted.

capnography the process of measuring and obtaining a tracing of the proportion of carbon dioxide in expired air using a capnograph.

carboxyhemoglobin hemoglobin on which the sites for oxygen are bound with carbon monoxide molecules.

cardiac output the amount of blood pumped from the heart in one minute; cardiac output equals stroke volume times heart rate.

chest physical therapy (CPT) a collection of therapeutic techniques designed to facilitate clearance of airway secretions, improve the distribution of ventilation, and enhance the efficiency and conditioning of the muscles of respiration; techniques include positioning, chest percussion and vibration, directed coughing, and various breathing and conditioning exercises.

chief complaint a subjective statement made by the patient describing the most significant sign or symptom of illness or dysfunction.

chlorofluorocarbons Freon propellants used in MDIs.

cilia hairlike processes that extend from a cell surface.

circumoral around the mouth.

compliance the relative ease with which a body stretches or deforms; in pulmonary physiology, a measure of volume change per unit pressure under static conditions (ml/cmH_2O); the reciprocal of elastance.

conscious awake and alert; aware of one's external environment.

consolidation the process of becoming solid; seen in the lung with certain types of pneumonia from the collection of exudate and loss of aeration.

continuous flow a constant flow of gas delivered during the inspiratory and expiratory phases of breathing.

contractility the ability of a muscle to become short in response to a stimulus.

contraindication a factor that prohibits the administration of a drug or performance of a procedure in the care of a patient.

corticosteroid any of the natural or synthetic hormones associated with the adrenal cortex.

crackles discontinuous type of lung sound heard on auscultation of the chest, usually during inspiration; formerly called rales.

crepitus producing a dry, crackling sound.

croup an acute viral infection of the upper respiratory tract that occurs primarily in infants and young children 3 months to 3 years of age after an upper respiratory infection; characterized by hoarseness, fever, a distinctive harsh, brassy cough, persistent stridor during inspiration, and varying degrees of respiratory distress resulting from obstruction of the larynx.

cyanosis bluish discoloration of the skin or mucous membranes caused by desaturation of at least 5 grams of hemoglobin per 100 ml of arterial blood.

deadspace gas volume that does not participate in gas exchange; three types include anatomic, alveolar, and physiologic.

dehydration a condition that results from undue loss of water.

depolarization the reduction of a membrane's resting potential to a less negative value.

diaphoresis profuse perspiration.

digitalis a cardiotonic drug.

diplococcus a spherical bacterium usually occurring in pairs.

dry powder inhaler (DPI) a small apparatus containing a unit dose of powdered drug for inhalation.

dyspnea subjective sensation of difficulty in breathing.

edema accumulation of excess fluid.

elastic capable of resuming its normal shape after distention.

electrocardiogram a record of the electrical activity of the heart; also known as ECG and EKG.

emphysema a chronic pulmonary disease in which there is destruction of the terminal bronchioles and air spaces leading to permanent enlargement that results in obstruction to airflow, air trapping, and gas exchange abnormalities.

endotracheal tube an artificial airway catheter that can be inserted into the trachea during endotracheal intubation to assure patency of the upper airway.

FEV_1 forced expiratory volume in one second; the volume of gas exhaled in the first second during a forced vital capacity maneuver.

FEV_1/FVC the ratio of forced expiratory volume in the first second to the total forced vital capacity volume expressed as a percentage.

fibrosis formation of fibrous tissue.

flowmeter a device used to measure the rate of flow of gases and liquids.

flow sheet a patient care record used to document interventions and patient response and condition.

flow volume loop a graphic analysis of the flow generated during forced vital capacity and forced inspiratory volume maneuvers plotted against volume change.

furosemide a loop diuretic used to treat edema and hypertension.

forced expiratory flow 25%-75% (FEF$_{25\%-75\%}$) the average flowrate during the middle half of an FVC curve.

forced expiratory volume (FEV) volume of gas expired over a given time interval from the beginning of a forced vital capacity maneuver.

forced vital capacity (FVC) maximum volume of gas that can be exhaled when the subject exhales forcefully and rapidly after a maximal inspiration.

fremitus a tremulous vibration of the chest wall that can be auscultated or palpated during physical examination.

gastric lavage irrigation or washing out of the stomach.

goblet cells mucus-producing cells.

gram-positive refers to the retention of stain in the Gram's method of staining for identification of bacteria.

hematocrit the percentage, by volume, of packed cells in a blood sample, expressed as a percentage.

hemoglobin protein molecule of the red blood cell that transports oxygen.

hemothorax blood in the pleural space.

hyperinflation therapy modalities used in respiratory therapy, such as incentive spirometry, intermittent positive pressure breathing (IPPB) therapy, and breathing exercises; to facilitate hyperinflation of the lungs, thereby preventing or reversing atelectasis; also helps the patient produce an effective cough and aids in the removal of secretions.

hyperpnea deep breathing.

hypertension increased blood pressure.

hyperresonance an increase in resonance.

hyperventilation ventilation in excess of that necessary to meet metabolic needs; signified by a PaCO$_2$ less than 35 mm Hg (torr) in the arterial blood.

hypotension low blood pressure.

hypoventilation ventilation less than that which is necessary to meet metabolic needs; signified by a PaCO$_2$ greater than 45 mm Hg (torr) in arterial blood.

hypoxemia a deficiency of oxygen in the arterial blood.

hypoxia an abnormal condition in which there is not enough oxygen available to the body's cells.

idiopathic occurring with no known cause.

incentive spirometry a breathing exercise using a device to accomplish a sustained maximal inspiration that mimics a natural sigh.

infection a disease caused by the invasion of the body by pathogenic microorganisms.

infection control the policies and procedures of a health-care facility to minimize the risk of nosocomial or community-acquired infections spreading to patients or members of the staff.

infrared (light) electromagnetic radiation with wavelengths between 10^{-5} and 10^{-4} meters; perceived as heat when it strikes the body.

inspection visual examination of the patient.

inspiratory capacity (IC) the maximum amount of air that can be inhaled from the resting end-expiratory level of functional residual capacity; the sum of tidal volume and inspiratory reserve volume.

intermittent positive pressure breathing (IPPB) the application of positive pressure breaths, usually with accompanying humidity or aerosol therapy, to a spontaneously breathing patient as a short-term treatment modality; usually provided for periods of time not exceeding 15 to 20 minutes.

intravenous within a vein; usually describing a method for infusing fluids or drugs.

intubation the passage of a tube into a body aperture; commonly refers to the insertion of an endotracheal tube within the trachea.

ischemia a localized reduction in perfusion to a body organ or part; often marked by pain and organ dysfunction, as in ischemic heart disease.

larynx the muscular and cartilaginous structure of the upper airway containing the vocal cords; lined with mucous membrane and sits below the root of the tongue and above the trachea; it is commonly called the voice box.

lethargy a condition of abnormal drowsiness or stupor.

mean mass aerodynamic diameter (MMAD) the distribution of aerosol particle diameter around which the mass of the particles is equally distributed with 50% of the particles heavier and 50% lighter.

mechanical ventilation the application of positive pressure at the airway opening during every inspiration to assist patients who are unable to adequately oxygenate or ventilate spontaneously.

mediastinum the area between the sternum and vertebral column containing the heart, large vessels, trachea, esophagus, thymus, and lymph nodes.

metered dose inhaler (MDI) a pressurized cartridge used for self-administration of exact dosages of aerosolized drugs; a type of self-propelled device designed to self-administer exact dosage of a concentrated medication.

methemoglobin a compound formed from hemoglobin by oxidation of the iron atom to the ferric state; does not function as an oxygen carrier and is present in the blood in small amounts.

morphine a narcotic analgesic and respiratory depressant.

mucociliary pertaining to ciliated mucosa.

myocardial infarction necrosis of the cells of an area of the heart muscle occurring as a result of ischemia and oxygen deprivation; commonly referred to as a "heart attack."

narcotic a drug that produces insensibility or stupor.

obesity excessive accumulation of fat in the body.

obstruction something that blocks or clogs and prevents passage.

osteoporosis condition of decreased volume of mineralized bone compared to age- and sex-matched controls.

overdose an excessive dose.

oximetry the process of determining the saturation of hemoglobin with oxygen using an oximeter.

oxygen a tasteless, odorless, colorless gas that is essential for human respiration.

oxygen therapy any procedure in which oxygen is administered to a patient to relieve hypoxia or hypoxemia.

oxyhemoglobin saturation the amount of oxygen actually combined with hemoglobin; expressed as a percentage of the oxygen capacity of that hemoglobin.

palpation the technique used in physical examination in which the examiner uses the hands or fingers to feel the texture, size, consistency, and location of certain parts of the patient's body.

past medical history an overall summary of the patient's general health to date including past injuries, allergies, surgical procedures, immunizations, hospitalizations, and obstetric and psychiatric history.

pathophysiology the study of biological and physical manifestations of a disease.

patient assessment an examiner's evaluation of a patient's disease or condition based on the patient's subjective report of the symptoms and course of the illness or condition, as well as the examiner's objective findings, including data obtained through laboratory tests, physical examination, and medical history.

patient interview a systematic questioning of a patient to obtain information that can be used to develop an individualized plan for care.

peak expiratory flow (PEF) maximum flow attained during a forced vital capacity maneuver.

peak inspiratory pressure the highest pressure that occurs during inspiration while on mechanical positive pressure ventilation/support.

pedal pertaining to the feet.

pediatric pertaining to the treatment of children and the study of childhood diseases.

penicillin antibiotic derived directly or indirectly from strains of fungi of the genus *Penicillium* and other soil-inhabiting fungi grown on special culture media.

percussion a technique of physical examination that involves striking the finger of one hand on a finger of the other as it is placed over the lung to discover the presence of air or fluid in the lungs.

perfusion the passage of a fluid such as blood through a specific organ or an area of the body.

pH shorthand notation that describes the hydrogen ion (H+) activity or hydrogen ion concentration in a solution; pH is usually expressed to the second decimal point (7.40).

physical examination the process of examining a patient for physical signs of disease or disorder.

pigment any organic coloring material produced by or introduced into the body.

plasma the fluid portion of the blood.

plateau pressure the pressure measured at the proximal airway during an end-inspiratory pause; a reflection of alveolar pressure.

pleura the serous membrane covering the lungs and lining the thoracic cavity, forming a potential space called the pleural space.

pleural effusion abnormal collection of fluid in the pleural space.

pleuritic pertaining to the pleura.

***Pneumocystis carinii* pneumonia** an acute interstitial plasma cell pneumonia characterized by a slight increase in fever, nonproductive cough, tachypnea, and dyspnea; caused by *Pneumocystis carinii*, an organism thought to be a protozoan; usually associated with patients with HIV disease who are severely immunocompromised.

pneumococcus an individual organism of the species *Streptococcus pneumoniae*; a common cause of lobar pneumonia.

pneumonia an inflammatory process of the lung parenchyma, usually infectious in origin.

pneumothorax the presence of air or gas in the pleural space of the thorax; called a tension pneumothorax if the air or gas is trapped under pressure.

positive expiratory pressure (PEP) mask therapy the application and maintenance of pressure above atmospheric at the airway throughout the expiratory phase of breathing; used as a bronchial hygiene technique to help mobilize secretions.

positive end-expiratory pressure (PEEP) the application and maintenance of pressure above atmospheric at the airway throughout the expiratory phase of positive pressure mechanical ventilation.

pressure support pressure-limited, assisted ventilation.

pulmonary pertaining to the lungs or respiratory system.

pulmonary edema accumulation of fluid in the tissues and air spaces of the lungs.

pulse oximetry the noninvasive estimation of arterial oxyhemoglobin saturation based on the combined principles of photoplethysmography and spectrophotometry.

pursed-lip breathing respiration characterized by deep inspirations followed by prolonged expirations through pursed lips.

purulent containing or forming pus.

refractory nonresponsive.

repolarization the process by which the cell is restored to its resting potential.

resonance a moderately low-pitched sound produced by percussion of an organ or cavity of the body during physical examination.

respiratory acidosis acidosis resulting from ventilation impairment and subsequent retention of CO_2, leading to an accumulation of the H+ ion concentration and lowered pH.

respiratory alkalosis alkalosis resulting from reduced CO_2 tension in the blood caused by hyperventilation, leading to a reduced H+ ion concentration and elevated pH.

respiratory rate the rate of breathing; normally 12 to 20 breaths per minute at rest.

SA node sinoatrial node, the pacemaker of the heart.

shunt ($\dot{Q}s/\dot{Q}t$) a bypass; as applied to cardiovascular and pulmonary medicine, an actual or physiologic connection between the right (venous) and left (arterial) sides of circulation.

sign an objective finding as perceived by the examiner.

small-volume nebulizer (SVN) a device that contains a volume of less than 30 milliliters of liquid and produces an aerosol from the volume contained; primarily used for short-term medication delivery to patients.

spacer an accessory device used with an MDI to reduce oropharyngeal medication deposition and reduce or eliminate the need for hand-breath coordination.

spirogram graphic display of lung volumes and capacities.

symptoms a subjective indication of a disease or change in condition as perceived by the examiner.

synchronized intermittent mandatory ventilation (SIMV) periodic assisted ventilation with positive pressure, which allows the patient to breathe spontaneously between breaths.

tachycardia a heart rate over 100 beats per minute.

tachypnea an abnormally rapid rate of breathing.

tidal volume (VT) the amount of air inhaled and exhaled during normal ventilation.

total lung capacity (TLC) the total amount of gas in the lungs after a maximum inspiration.

tuberculosis (TB) a reportable infectious disease caused by *Mycobacterium tuberculosis*, usually chronic in nature, and commonly affecting the lungs although it may occur in almost any part of the body.

T-piece (Briggs adapter) a device used with artificial airways that has two 22 mm adapters opposite each other and a 15 mm port at right angles forming a T; attached to large bore aerosol tubing and a nebulizer to provide a continuous flow of aerosol to the bypassed airway.

vesicular breath sounds a normal sound of air movement as detected during auscultation of the chest; characteristically higher in pitch during inspiration and fading rapidly during expiration.

viscosity the resistance to flow.

vital capacity (VC) the total amount of air that can be exhaled after a maximum inspiration; the sum of the inspiratory reserve volume, tidal volume, and the expiratory reserve volume.

vocal fremitus the vibration of the chest wall as a person speaks, allowing the person's voice to be heard by the examiner during auscultation of the chest with a stethoscope.

wheeze a sound heard on auscultation of the chest characterized by a high-pitched, musical quality.